RADICAL
RECOVERY

RADICAL RECOVERY

*Extraordinary Healing
with* OXYGEN *&* LIGHT *After
Chemo and Radiation*

EDNA NESS

NEW YORK

LONDON • NASHVILLE • MELBOURNE • VANCOUVER

Radical Recovery

Extraordinary Healing with Oxygen & Light After Chemo and Radiation

Published in New York, New York, by Morgan James Publishing in partnership with Difference Press. Morgan James is a trademark of Morgan James, LLC. www.MorganJamesPublishing.com.

The Morgan James Speakers Group can bring authors to your live event. For more information or to book an event visit The Morgan James Speakers Group at www.TheMorganJamesSpeakersGroup.com.

ISBN 9781683508212 paperback
ISBN 9781683508229 eBook
Library of Congress Control Number: 2017916534

Cover Design by:
Rachel Lopez
www.r2cdesign.com

Interior Design by:
Chris Treccani
www.3dogcreative.net

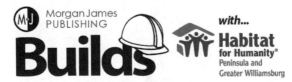

In an effort to support local communities, raise awareness and funds, Morgan James Publishing donates a percentage of all book sales for the life of each book to Habitat for Humanity Peninsula and Greater Williamsburg.

Get involved today! Visit
www.MorganJamesBuilds.com

Dedication

I dedicate this book to my parents who loved me
unconditionally
and gave me the heart and desire to serve others, and
to my soulmate Douglas for choosing to stay on this earth a
little longer;
for working hard to learn and grow through your healing
journey;
for opening your heart to unlimited unconditional love;
for changing my life and being my hero.

Table of Contents

Introduction

I wrote this book in hopes of helping others find healing after the damaging effects of chemo and radiation treatments. The American Medical Association has a "standard of care" for treating cancer, but in my experience there is no "standard of care" to recover and heal afterward. My husband's case was extreme, and his healing outcome was extraordinary.

Our Story

My husband and I were struggling in our marriage and were in the middle of a move. We were hooking up our new washer and dryer when I got a 220-volt shock that should have killed me. It left me with roaming electrical pain, nerve damage to my right arm, and caused my already chronic migraines to intensify. This shock would change our lives forever in ways we never could have imagined.

Having worked in natural healing for over 10 years at the time, I already knew about hyperbaric oxygen therapy. After the electrical shock and thinking I may never be able to work again, I bought a mild hyperbaric chamber for home use and combined it with the light therapy I had already been using for a decade. Not only had I been using light therapy personally, I was also in the process of building a business that focused on selling these systems to practitioners and home users. I had recently gained a business partner and we were in the midst of bringing it all together when I was injured. Seeking out hyperbaric oxygen therapy was already on our radar, and I felt that this synergistic approach would get me the healing I needed. If I was granted my healing, I would open a healing center to offer hyperbaric services and educate others about the rejuvenating power of oxygen and light. If I didn't get my healing, I would sell the chamber and keep searching.

To my surprise, this was *not only* the answer to repair my nerve damage from the electric shock, but also for the chronic migraines I had suffered from for 30 years. This was a miracle!

Four months later, I followed through on the commitment I made to myself. I opened In Light Hyperbarics, a place for hope and healing. I wanted to share my newfound miracle with others who needed healing, not knowing at the time that God had a bigger plan.

We had no way of knowing, but God was giving us the gift of a lifetime. We would both have life-threatening situations nine months apart. I, with my electrical shock, and nine months later my husband, Doug, with advanced stage IV throat cancer. We were in a time of crisis and would have to put our differences aside and fight for our lives.

Our relationship continued to struggle as he didn't really understand why I spent money on this equipment and he did not share my passion for helping others. Little did he know, it would become his lifeline as well. Doug was diagnosed three months after opening my business. Everything happened so fast, as if time sped up and came to a screeching halt all at once. I remember thinking that life as we knew it was over. I would learn how to be strong during one of the darkest times of my life, and my husband would eventually become a changed man through it all. He had to have 33 radiation and two very large chemo treatments. He recovered, but emerged from treatment a broken, damaged man with a broken spirit. How could I allow this to be his "new normal" following treatment? His life was saved, but his health and vitality suffered.

I had to walk away from my business, but I was blessed with the opportunity to guide my husband through the recovery and healing that gave him a second chance at life, and us a second chance at love. These struggles have given me knowledge, confidence, and tons of experience using oxygen and light to support the human body and accelerate the healing process. His case was extreme and his healing outcome was extraordinary. His recovery was something the doctors never thought possible. They called it a miracle.

God had a plan, and His plan was a perfect plan.

This book was part of His plan, to help others know there is a way to have radical healing after radical cancer treatment. For those of you reading this book, it is my hope and prayer that you also get your second chance; that you break away from your prison of pain with a more complete healing. I welcome you into the stories of others who have trusted my guidance. Those who made the commitment to give mild hyperbaric oxygen and light therapy the opportunity to help alleviate their pain and restore their health. If you are suffering from the ravages of cancer treatment, I encourage you to keep reading and learn how you, too, can shine through the darkness of pain and disease.

CHAPTER 1

You Never Know Until You Know; Our Journey

"All the flowers of tomorrow are in the seeds of today."
– Indian Proverb

Begin with the End in Mind

Doug's life became a nightmare overnight. One day he was in Key West for the boat races, having a great time hanging out with friends, and a few days later he was in Vancouver, WA where he was diagnosed with stage IV throat cancer. He had a massive tumor in the base of his tongue that was preparing to choke him, and surgery was not an option. He needed 33 daily radiation and three very large chemotherapy treatments.

At the end of two months, every inch of his throat and mouth were blistered from the radiation. This is all a blur to him, since he was in what I called a "walking coma" from an overdose sustained in the hospital.

He was unable to swallow and had to use a suction machine so he wouldn't choke on his own saliva and phlegm. He was on a feeding tube for his meals, hydration, and medication. His pain was excruciating; he was on high doses of opiates that caused severe constipation and kept him sedated. He had chemo brain on top of brain trauma from the overdose of opiates. He was not able to communicate very well, and he had high levels of anxiety and depression.

He was having problems with orthostatic hypotension: his blood pressure dropped when he stood up, which caused him to faint. He could not be left alone and needed help with every function of his life. His healing prognosis was grim. He would most likely never regain his swallowing or full use of his tongue, taste buds, salivary glands, or jaw. There was a good chance his neck would develop thick scar tissue, limiting his neck and facial movement. Radiation destroys bone and its blood supply which can over time cause osteoradionecrosis. This means his jaw bone would begin to deteriorate and basically cause his face to fall apart. These are all the physical problems he was facing, which doesn't touch all the lifestyle, emotional, and relationship problems that were included in this nightmare. This was not the way he pictured his life in the golden years: How would he ever make it through this pain, destruction and sadness? How would he ever rebuild his body to have some quality of life?

He made it through this nightmare because of a fateful decision he made many years ago. He met a woman who was kind, caring and a little different from the other women he had dated. She was attentive, a good listener and was always trying to make sure everyone around her was taken care of. *He fell in love with her heart*, but it troubled him that she loved helping others to a fault. She would put others' needs in front of her own; she wanted to serve everyone. But on the other hand, that is why he loved her. This woman he fell in love with was me.

I was meant to be here to help him. I was sent to care for him in his darkest hours. I would lift him up, bring him light, love and hope. I would be given the knowledge throughout my life to guide him through his healing; to be there for him, to put his needs in front of my own.

This was God's plan. His plan to touch his heart to make him a better man and us a stronger couple. His plan to further my ability to help and nurture others in pain and healing. To have the awareness and expertise to assist those people suffering with cancer and the devastating effects from traditional treatment.

A Bleak Prognosis

Doug was diagnosed with stage IV base-of-tongue squamous cell carcinoma on December 3, 2014. We began the long journey to figure out what treatment he needed and who would be the best team of doctors for him. I was frantically doing my research to gain knowledge about tongue cancer. The more I learned about throat cancer and the devastating effects of radiation and chemotherapy, the more concerned I became about whether he would want to live with the collateral damage. After reading many discussion groups of others who had gone through head and neck cancer, it was clear to me that the prognosis and long-term effects were not pretty. In fact, they were ugly, completely depressing and horrific in many cases. Here are a few of the long-term effects he would possibly face but didn't want to hear about:

- Loss of the ability to swallow
- Loss of voice
- Limited use of jaw
- Loss of taste buds
- Loss of saliva glands
- Severe burning from radiation
- Long-term scar tissue that would limit ability to turn neck
- Vein damage
- Chemo brain

The potential devastation was shocking to me. There were many people in the discussion groups that were still on a feeding tube 10 years after treatment. The most devastating side effect was that the radiation would kill the bone marrow in his jaw and he would no longer have blood flow to that area of his face. Osteoradionecrosis could set in, and his jaw would start to deteriorate. The more I learned, the more concerned I became. I wanted to share the information with him, but *he* didn't want to know. He held on to the fact that *I would fix him* in the end and knew that it was my passion to help others to heal. *This would be a tall order and new territory for me!*

Looking for Alternatives: X-Ray Radiation or Proton Therapy

Looking back, it's clear that it was the fear of the unknown that fueled my fire to do everything I could. I was well aware that his life would never be the same again. I was on a warpath to find the best mainstream cancer center in the country with the best doctors. I was looking for alternative radiation therapy that would not leave him so damaged. That's when I discovered proton therapy, a different type of radiation that doesn't have the devastating effects of X-ray radiation. There are only 12 proton treatment centers in America, and we're lucky enough to have one in Seattle. I knew we were running against the clock, but I felt we needed to look at proton radiation as an option.

As I was frantically making calls and pulling together his records to see if proton radiation was an option for him, we continued to move through the process of showing up to his appointments and meeting the teams of doctors to determine where to have treatment. I was not impressed with our choice of doctors. It seemed to me that Doug was just a number to them, and it was more about themselves, not about his suffering and fighting for his life. Our family was feeling apprehensive about me continuing to search for other options. I understood they just wanted to get him in for treatment *now*! I also was taking this very seriously. This was *his life* and this was the *choice of a lifetime, the choice about his life moving forward and the quality of that life!*

Second-Guessing the Doctors

It seemed that the doctors didn't really like it when I asked them questions,especially when it came to diet, alternative care and proton therapy. In their opinion, they felt he should eat anything he wanted—including sugar—to keep weight on throughout treatment. It was my opinion that sugar feeds the tumor, so he should stay away from it. I wanted him on a healthy diet to protect his healthy cells as much as possible, cleanse, and detoxify the body. Also, since they didn't offer proton therapy, they clearly didn't see it as an option. What I came to realize was that, if they don't offer a particular treatment, they really don't know much about it. They took offense that I would second-guess their treatment options. Time was running out; it was time to make a choice where he would have treatment. Doug chose to have his simulation done at Providence Hospital in Portland, Oregon. His appointment would be the following Monday.

To my surprise, I received a call from Seattle Cancer Care Alliance with a scheduled consultation the following Tuesday, the day after his simulation. My hopes were still high for him to be considered for proton therapy and to have him accepted into the Seattle program. It was a long shot and I had no idea how we would make it work, but I wanted the best for him.

A Turn for the Worse; Tumor Ulceration

It was Friday, three days before he would go in for his simulation. His pain was more than he could bear when swallowing, and he felt that something had changed on the side of his tongue. Sure enough, he now had a marble sized ulcerated lump coming out the right side of his tongue. I called the hospital and they said the doctor would look at it when he came in on Monday. I had a feeling it was the tumor, but I wasn't sure. He was no longer able to swallow without excruciating pain so eating was not an option. The tumor was sitting on his facial nerve, so even swallowing his own saliva was painful. It was a helpless feeling for all of us.

This week would be a turning point. He would have the simulation done at Providence Monday morning and Tuesday morning we would drive to Seattle for a consultation at the University of Washington Medical Center. I was amazed, after all of the appointments with all of the doctors, that no one had given us any inkling of how long he had to live. They all just seemed to be going through the motions at their own pace without a worry. Is that how it's supposed to be?

Where Does Empathy Play a Role?

Monday morning, we arrived for his simulation. As the doctor examined his mouth, he confirmed that the tumor had now come through the wall of his tongue and was ulcerated. It was getting in the way of his teeth closing, so he was no longer able to talk. I asked the doctor if he could give him something for the pain. He went to the cupboard to grab a topical ointment. I was bewildered as he rubbed a small amount on the ulcerated lump. It did nothing for his pain. The following conversation would shock and anger me for the rest of my life, and quite frankly, I hope it haunts the doctor for the rest of his:

> *Doctor:* Stop at the store on your way home for some Anbesol *(over-the counter ointment used for teething).*
> *Me:* Is there anything else you could give him for pain?

Doctor: No, try the Anbesol first.

Me: OK… I think we should schedule a time to have a feeding tube placed.

Doctor: I don't like to start my patients with a feeding tube before starting treatment.

Me: But he can't swallow anymore, and he hasn't eaten for three days.

Doctor: (looks at Doug in a stern way): Just swallow!

Wow, where does empathy play a role in cancer treatment? Obviously, we were in the wrong place for warmth and compassion. We were stunned! You want to put trust in your doctor and feel he is doing what's right. You want to believe he truly cares. This was not the feeling I got from that doctor.

I was so puzzled; why would they not help him? I had a sick feeling in my stomach as I tried to coax Doug to drink a nutritional shake. Now, I was more anxious than ever to get to Seattle for his consultation. All we could do was pray for more empathy, compassion and a better team of doctors willing to take fast action.

A Week to Live

There we were, sitting in a treatment room at University of Washington Medical Center. Doug had become so weak from not eating, and he now carried a white board for communication. The door opened and Dr. A walked in, introduced himself, and when he looked at Doug, his face turned to the most compassionate, empathic expression I've ever seen on a doctor. He tilted his head and said, "Oh my gosh, you are in so much pain. I'm so sorry." *Wow!* No one needed to tell him how much pain Doug was in, and he saw him as a human, not a number! I knew at that moment we were in the right place. *This is what cancer care should feel like.*

Dr. A proceeded to explain to us that Doug would have been a good candidate for proton therapy, but we didn't have enough time. The planning time for proton therapy takes about three weeks, and he was concerned that he would not survive through the weekend. *Wow, he was telling us that Doug only had less than a week to live!* We are a bit shocked—but grateful—that someone was willing to give us a time frame. *Dr. A was actually honest with us!*

Dr. A explained that if Doug wanted to have treatment in Seattle they would do his simulation right away. They would put a Fentanyl pain patch on his arm and give him another pain medication for his spikes of pain. He would work overtime to get the radiation plan done so that Doug could begin treatment by the following Tuesday. He said they would schedule surgery ASAP to place a feeding tube. Wow, again! *Dr. A is actually trying to save his life!*

Jumping Through Hoops

It was a big decision to have treatment in Seattle away from home, but we all knew we were in the right place. The cancer center was rated fourth in the nation, the doctor showed compassion and empathy, and they were jumping through hoops to save his life. Dr. A's nurse, Angela, was short and tiny—but she took charge. I didn't know it at the time, but she would end up playing a very large part in saving Doug's life and helping me through the next two months. She was an angel sent from God. There was absolutely no question we were in the right place. What a contrast to what we had been dealing with for the last month.

The following morning, we met with Dr. B at the Seattle Cancer Care Alliance: She would be his medical oncologist. She was a woman of grace. She didn't wear a white coat like most doctors. Her attire was elegant; she wore beautiful dresses with a classy style. She carried herself with charm and expressed as much compassion and empathy as Dr. A had.

It was in her office that we got the first look at the tumor from a PET scan. It is a memory that will forever be etched in my mind: the image of this monstrous tumor that was living inside of him. I stood in shock. How could anyone live with this in their throat and not know it for so long? As I stared at the screen, the tumor glowing in bright yellow, Dr. B's phone rang and after a brief consultation with Dr. A she informed us that they put a rush on his treatment in hopes of saving his life. "Your feeding tube will be placed on Friday so you can finally have a meal," she said. We were more relieved and even more confident that we had made the right decision to come to Seattle. The whole family was praying for Doug.

CHAPTER 2

Truly a Life Saving Trip

"You can only go halfway into the darkest forest; then you are
coming out the other side."
– Chinese Proverb

Life Was Slipping Away

We arrived in Seattle on Tuesday morning, and it was now Friday. We had been staying at a hotel while we looked for a small apartment to call home for the next several months during Doug's treatment. He had a really rough first night and could no longer lay down without choking. His breathing had become very labored and I could hear a gurgling sound deep in his throat which told me the tumor had grown. It had been one week since his last meal and he had had minimal fluids. He was extremely weak and his skin was pale with a hint of gray. This told me he wasn't getting enough oxygen. This was going to be a big day: he would be having surgery for the feeding tube placement.

I felt so grateful that we would finally be able to feed him. I was so scared for him but trying to keep my spirits up. I hadn't had much sleep myself, as I spent much of the night making sure Doug was still breathing. My heart was heavy. I was so grateful to have the love and support of our daughters around us, as we couldn't have managed without them.

We checked Doug in at the Digestive Disease Center at the University of Washington Medical Center on January 8, 2014. The doctor came into the room to clear him for surgery preparation, but he left without saying much. Soon he returned with a team of doctors, and they all squeezed into the small exam room. You could feel the tension and apprehension; I knew in my heart it was not good news. They informed us that they would not be able to place the feeding tube as the tumor had grown since his last examination. They could not safely thread the tube down his throat without suffocating him. To safely place the tube, they would need an operating room and there wasn't one available until the following Wednesday. *That was five days from now.* As the doctors filed out of the room, we were devastated. I could see the fear in Doug's eyes. The hope of living through this nightmare was slipping away. He was starving to death and would soon suffocate. It was hard to hide my own fear and sadness.

A Doctor Plays God with Opiates

Feeling helpless and in disbelief, I called the oncology radiation department to get advice on what we should do now. The intern explained to us that they were unable to admit him into the hospital—but that's what needed to happen. Doug was not going to live another night without having fluids. She instructed us to take him to the emergency room and have him admitted for a *pain evaluation*. This would allow him to be hooked up to an IV for fluids and to administer pain meds. So, off to the ER we went.

What a difference a bag of fluids can make to a dying man. Within 24 hours, he had color in his face and no longer looked like he was on the brink of death. He was still in a lot of pain and hungry as all get out, but he was finally able to rest a little better knowing he would be getting some care. He still had the 25mg Fentanyl patch on his arm for continuous pain relief, but they also put him on morphine for the spikes of pain. By Saturday evening, the morphine was making him sick to his stomach, so they switched it to 4 mils of Dilaudid. I wasn't familiar with opiates, so I put my complete trust in the doctors.

That morning our oldest daughter left to go back to her family in Portland so I was now alone with Doug. Our other daughters had found a small furnished apartment for us to live in for the next few months, and it was just 10 minutes from the hospital. They were in the process of moving our things over from the hotel and filling the cupboards with food. We had decided that it was my job to take care of their father and their job to make sure that I ate. What a blessing! Early Sunday morning Doug woke up in a terrible panic—he wanted out of that hospital bed. I took him for a short walk down the hallway, and after several rounds he was willing to go back to the room and sit on the bench by the window. He held onto me so tight I could tell he didn't want to leave me, and that he was afraid of dying. With that look of terror in his eyes, he couldn't talk and he couldn't express his feelings but I knew what he was thinking. He could hardly breathe. Tears began to fall down his face. I felt so helpless, all I could do was love him, hold him and pray for him to have peace.

After a couple of hours I was finally able to get him to lay down with me in the bed. Before long the doctor came in and sat next to the bed. She explained that it was no longer necessary for us to be in the hospital, so she would be ordering his release and sending the nurse in with the new medications. I was dumbfounded; if there was ever a time that Doug needed to be in the hospital, it was now. But as I mentioned, I was putting my trust in the doctors so I tried to be positive about it with him.

The nurse came in with his new medication. She had a handful of syringes full of a red liquid and a new 50mg Fentanyl patch for his arm. The syringes were filled with liquid Dilaudid. The nurse explained that the new prescription would be 8 mils of Dilaudid every three hours and a new 50mg Fentanyl patch every 72 hours. They had ordered his release and someone would be in to get us soon. So, they had just doubled his opiates and were going to send him home with me.

Barely a Heartbeat

I asked for some towels and supplies so that I could give Doug a shower before we left, and the nurse accommodated us but gave no assistance. After getting him cleaned up and dressed, I laid next to him in the bed as we awaited the chariot. With my head on his chest, listening to his labored breathing, I started to count our breaths. For every four of mine, he had one. I began watching the clock and realized he was taking only four breaths a minute. I knew this wasn't right, but I didn't know what to do. I was trusting the doctors, because I didn't know about throat cancer or opiates, and they did. They never came back in the room to check his vitals before we left.

In hindsight, I should have never taken him out of the hospital, and they should not have released him. He was opiate naïve; he had only been on opiates for five days. They should have observed Doug for at least 24 hours after increasing his opiates. They should not have increased two different opiates at the same time, let alone double both of them at once.

It took me about 6-8 months to realize it, but I believe this doctor had been playing God. She thought she was doing us a favor by overdosing him and sending him home with me to die. *Little did she know I was not going to let that happen on my watch.*

A Long, Lonely Night

I took Doug home to our new little apartment, a perfect place for us to be at the time. All I needed to do was focus on him. I could tell immediately that he was overdosed. As I tried coaxing him to drink small bits of a nutritional shake, he would go into a trance and hold it in his mouth without swallowing. I had to keep reminding him over and over and over again to *"Just swallow, Douglas, just swallow, sweetheart, just swallow."* I couldn't leave his side.

I was afraid to let him sleep and had to continually prompt him to breathe all through the night. I made the fateful decision to not give him the doses of Dilaudid he had been prescribed. Oh my, he was so out of it. He began to hallucinate, he was seeing other people in the room and also stayed busy with his hands as if he was working or hanging things up. I had to stay focused on the fact that his radiation treatments were going to start tomorrow, chemo would start on Tuesday, and Wednesday he would finally get his feeding tube. I was so exhausted, but if

I could just hold myself together and keep him alive for three more days, maybe, just maybe, he would live through this and beat the odds. I so badly needed to sleep, but that would have to wait another day. I prayed, talked to God, talked to my parents in Heaven and continued to just give him love.

Radiation Begins

It was Monday morning. He made it through the night and I was trying to get us both ready to head to the hospital for radiation. I only gave him one-half the dose of the prescribed Dilaudid early that morning and he was still so sedated that he couldn't do anything on his own. I had to dress him, help him to the bathroom, brush his teeth and help him from room to room. It felt like he was trying to decide whether to live or die. This was all so new to me; I've never seen anyone like this before. I didn't know how much of it was the medication, the cancer, the fear or the depression he had fallen into. I was just happy he was still breathing and we were on our way to his first radiation treatment.

Dr. A's nurse Angela came out to greet us. She would be my guardian angel at the hospital and help us get through the next two months. She walked us back through the winding hallways until we got to the dressing and radiation rooms. He wasn't able to walk on his own so I escorted him back and helped him get changed into a gown. They took us into the radiation room and it felt like something out of a horror film. They showed us his mask that was made during the simulation. The radiation machine was gigantic; it rotated around and around his head shooting beams of radiation to kill the tumor. The treatments were daily and lasted anywhere from 20 to 45 minutes. This is not something you want to go through if you are claustrophobic, and I knew he was! We had to give him Xanax an hour before each treatment so he wouldn't freak out.

I was so happy his treatment had started and they were just happy to see that Doug was still with us. I felt as though I should be mentioning something about his overdose from inpatient care on Sunday, but I still wasn't sure whether it was the cancer or the medication. I continued to just keep with the prescription schedule knowing that we would be back tomorrow. I was continually trying to get him to swallow little bits of shake for nutrition but it was a huge challenge. I gave him the Dilaudid, but only half the dose. The girls stopped by to give him some love and to make sure I was eating. We were all so glad he had started treatment and looked forward to him starting chemotherapy the next day. It was another long night of watching him breathe and not letting him slip away.

A Fall Down the Stairs

It was Tuesday, we had been in Seattle for one week, and Doug was holding on by a thread. We were gearing up for his second radiation treatment, followed by six hours of chemotherapy. He had a lot of hallucinations and panic attacks the night before. I could feel him slipping away, and it had now been 10 days since his last meal. While he was still in bed, I chopped off my hair. I just knew I needed to have my own grooming be fast and simple, and I didn't care what I looked like at this point. I was so exhausted and it was all I could do to get us both showered.

It was cold outside so I bundled him up and walked arm in arm out the front door. I had to let go of him for a moment and put down my bag while I locked the door behind us. I turned around to grab his arm and saw that, without me knowing, he had picked up the bag and was stepping off the top stair. My heart stopped as he started to fall. The weight of the bag miraculously spun him around as he was falling down the stairs, and it forced his arm to hook through the banister. It was like an angel was there to catch him. I was so grateful.

By the time I got him in the car and everything cleaned up, we were late. As we walked into the radiation department, I saw Angela's face and I burst into tears. She quickly ushered us back into a room and Dr. A followed.

They wanted to know what was wrong and what had happened with the pain evaluation during his inpatient stay. When they heard about the high doses of opiates and the fact that they had released us early without observing him, they were mortified. They decided it would be best to take him in for radiation and then wheel him down to the ER and re-admit him. Because of that fateful fall down the stairs they realized he was over sedated and in critical need of inpatient care and hydration.

CHAPTER 3

Chemo & Radiation Roller Coaster

"Never give up. This may be your moment for a miracle."
– Greg Anderson

The Critical 24 Hours

Here we go! The next 24 hours would be the turning point that would save his life. Our cancer team was not going to let anything stop them from giving him a second chance at life, and the hospital agreed to bend their rule of "no chemo as an in-patient." Here is the lifesaving rigid 24-hour schedule to save his life in this dire time:

January 13, 2015

2:00 p.m.—Radiation treatment #2

4:00 p.m.—Re-admit into the ER because of the overdose

Midnight to 6:00 a.m.—Chemotherapy

8:00 a.m.—Surgery for feeding tube placement

11:00 a.m.—Radiation treatment #3

After this brutal regimen, it was absolutely a miracle he was still with us. Hopefully, the tumor would begin to shrink and we would be able to feed him soon. I felt a small wave of relief wash over me. Dr. A and Dr. B kicked butt! They did everything possible to save his life. Our family is forever grateful!

Play by Play on the Roller Coaster

Over the next two months, Doug would continue to be in a sedated state. He was like a helpless child who couldn't think for himself, feed himself and he relied on me and our daughters for all of his needs. It would be a roller coaster of complications and close calls. In hindsight, it was the best decision for us to be far away from home, because our only focus was keeping him alive. Here is a timeline of the challenges he faced after his treatment started:

Week One

January 15: He had his first meal in 12 days. He was not out of the woods yet, but at least now we were able to get him the nutrition his body needed. To me, this was a game changer. Today we would learn how to feed him via the feeding tube, which was a big responsibility. We would have to start feeding small amounts and increase slowly, as it's a little uncomfortable to have food going directly into the stomach. Having a feeding tube placed was not something that either of us wanted for him, but now it was such a blessing.

January 16: He had a rough night and it seemed like he was having a hard time getting used to the food going into his stomach. Today would be his fifth radiation treatment, and then we would transport him by ambulance to the Specialty Dental Group to have his tongue splint made. This was in hopes of saving his tongue as much as possible from the radiation. This was not something that anyone in Portland ever mentioned, so I was pretty excited about anything that would help protect any part of his mouth from the radiation damage. They would create a mold of his tongue and make the splint while we were there, do a fitting, then make adjustments and fit it again and again. It was a long, hard appointment for him, and it would be his first time being fed out in public via the feeding tube. It was uncomfortable for both of us since we were both unsure and inexperienced.

January 19: This was day seven of radiation and he would be released from the hospital—but not without more complications. He hadn't had a bowel movement in 12 days. Although he hadn't eaten much, to me it was a major concern as he had been taking in a lot of toxins. Nonetheless, they released him into my care and it became another night of horror for him.

We were up all night, and he was in horrendous pain and full of fear. I was trying to figure out how to help him without taking him back to the hospital. All I can say is I am so grateful he doesn't even remember that specific night.

Week Two

January 20: With the help of our sweet nurse Angela, we were able to get a colon prep kit and guidance to hydrate his impacted intestinal tract from both ends. We were able to give him relief without putting him back in the hospital. From here on out I would watch his bowels like a hawk. I administered castor oil packs, heavy probiotics, aloe, lots of water through his tube and, once I got brave enough, we also added fiber via the tube. I had to be careful not to create a blockage in his tube. I also started him on a "whole food" feeding tube formula I found that would give him more nutrition and less sugar. The name of the food was so fitting: "Liquid Hope." It was literally our hope for healing!

January 22: This would be a great day! After ten days straight of radiation and a CT scan the day before, we met with Dr. A for his results. We knew that the tumor had shrunk because he was able to breathe more easily, and he could now talk and drink sips of water. The results were outstanding. Dr. A gave us the great news that the tumor reacted better than expected. He had never seen a tumor shrink so quickly. It had reduced in size so much that he would be revising his radiation program to minimize collateral damage. He also announced, "The voice you have today is the voice you should have at the end of treatment." We no longer had to worry about him suffocating from his tumor.

He was now in the "honeymoon stage" where the painful effects of radiation burns have not yet surfaced. Over the next week he would be able to eat small portions of normal food while continuing with his tube feedings. His weight had dropped from 175 to a low of 130. In the coming week he would gain back a mere three pounds, but every pound counted through this honeymoon stage!

Week Three

January 29: Dr. A did another simulation to scale down his treatment plan even further. We are so very grateful for him and his willingness to put in extra time and effort to reduce the collateral damage from the radiation. Tube feedings were going well and I felt we were finally on a good schedule. It was a challenge to figure out the right timing to get his four meals in, pushing water to stay hydrated and giving him the meds all through the tube. He wasn't able to lie down for two hours after I fed him because his meals tended to come right back up. It was a lot trickier than one might think, since he had to lie down for radiation treatments. Even though he was feeling better, he was still in a sedated state. He hadn't yet come out of it since the overdose and maybe that was the way God had planned it.

Week Four

February 2: On this day, he woke up with a very sore throat and was scheduled for a second round of chemotherapy. The honeymoon was over; he was no longer suffocating or starving, but he was beginning to burn inside and out from the damaging effects of the radiation. He no longer wanted to eat food via his mouth and would have to be prodded to swallow anything.

February 3: He was still battling with constipation due to the opiates, the chemotherapy drugs, the anti-nausea drugs, as well as the toxic effects from the radiation. This would be a constant battle even though we were going above and beyond to combat the problem.

This day he would also start a long battle with thrush, an oral infection caused by an overgrowth of candida. He had a creamy covering and small white bumps all over his tongue, inside of his cheeks and down his throat. This infection was very painful. Chemotherapy and radiation killed his healthy cells, which made him more susceptible to infections.

February7: At about 2 o'clock in the morning, I heard a thud and realized he was not in bed with me. I ran into the bathroom and there he was on the floor. He had fallen against the counter and scraped his chin. I helped him up and we headed towards the bedroom. I could feel him heading for the floor again, so I laid him down gently. This would be the beginning of a new complication called orthostatic hypotension and his body would have a hard time regulating its blood pressure. His blood pressure would be fine while laying down, but as soon as he sat or stood up it would drop dramatically causing him to faint. Once again, we would have to admit him into the hospital in an effort to figure out why this was happening.

Week Five

February 9: They released him from the hospital today because they couldn't find any reasons for the dramatic drop in his blood pressure. Hydration and anemia are big contributors to orthostatic hypotension, but those were not the problems he had. It was possible that he had some damage to the vagus nerve from the size of his tumor, so we had to watch him carefully, as well as have more testing done if the problem persisted. It was possible that his lack of exercise was a contributing factor, so we began forcing more movement.

February 10: At this point we were at a crossroads and we needed to get him moving to promote more oxygen flow to the brain. But he was so sedated that it was even hard to get him to walk to the edge of the driveway and back. In hind sight I wish we would have had one of our hyperbaric oxygen chambers with us, as it would have made such a big difference in so many ways. Doug's pain had increased due to the burning in his throat, but after much discussion, we decided it was time to remove his Fentanyl patch and try only giving him Dilaudid for pain relief. Maybe this decision would give him more energy to walk and help his blood pressure from dropping.

Week Six

February 17: Getting Doug off the Fentanyl patch was a good idea, as we were then able to keep him stable using only Dilaudid. However, exercise was still a continual struggle, along with the orthostatic hypotension. His throat and mouth were so blistered, inflamed and broken down that he needed to use a suction machine to help with the buildup of phlegm. We had him sleeping on the couch, sitting up, so that he wouldn't choke and he was unwilling and unable to swallow anything. I had to force him to swallow a tablespoon of aloe mixed with probiotics every two hours to keep his swallowing muscles working. I had been warned if you don't keep these muscles working, you might lose your ability to swallow in the future. He was not happy with me but I was not willing to let that happen to him.

February 23: This was his last radiation treatment, followed by what was supposed to be his last chemotherapy infusion. But tests showed that his white blood cell count was too low, and they told us he only had a 20% chance of living if we went through with it. Once again, he was fighting for his life. The days were long and hard, and it was so sad for all of us to watch him go through this.

February 24: We had been looking forward to this day for the last two months. It was his last visit with Dr. A before we headed home. We were grateful for his oncology team but we were so ready to begin the recovery process.

It was a strange feeling! To be so happy that treatment was completed, but also a little lost and in the dark about what lay ahead. Now what?

Holding On to Hope

The change in our daily routine left us feeling very empty. The last two months we had been going to the hospital daily for treatment and guidance. All of a sudden we were on our own to figure out how to heal him from the damage that was done by chemotherapy and radiation. These brutal treatments had saved his life and we were so thankful, but it didn't seem there was a "standard of care" for post treatment recovery. I had to continue to follow my intuition from all of my experiences with natural healing.

Through it all, I am so very grateful for my many years of working in the naturopathic field. I felt a deep appreciation for all the knowledge I gained from Dr. Heather and Dr. Rebecca about natural remedies and nutritional nourishment. I hope they know that their generosity, kindness, and the time they spent training me have gone to good use. Their voices led me through one of the darkest times of my life and gave me the strength to stay the course of doing anything and everything I could to protect Doug's healthy cells and reduce the side effects from his treatment. *I am forever grateful!*

Home at Last

Doug's last radiation treatment was on February 23, but he was too weak to make the trip home to Vancouver until March 12. As we made our way home, he was full of anxiety about seeing friends and family. How would they look at him? What would they think? He felt like a shell of the man that he used to be, and he couldn't even take care of himself. I reassured him that he didn't have to see anyone until he was ready. All that mattered now was that he was alive and coming home. Our loving family and friends just wanted to support us in his healing journey.

Due to the intense internal burns in his throat and mouth, he was still not able to lie flat. Our sons set up a recliner in the study and that is where he slept for the next couple of months.

He still relied on the feeding tube for all of his meals, hydration and meds as we helped him relearn how to swallow and eat.

Now, it was time for recovery! We moved one of the hyperbaric chambers home from my healing center and started giving him two one-hour sessions every day. This would prove to be one of the most important moves we made for his healing! Three months later we drove up to Seattle for his checkup. Dr. A was surprised at his fast recovery and to our delight he announced that Doug was already in remission! After only three months! He had never seen anything like it. The internal burns in his throat and mouth were healed, and there were no signs of scarring from the radiation or the tumor. The tissue in his throat was a beautiful pink color and it was working perfectly! After all we had been through, we were closer in our marriage than we had been in years and our love and appreciation for each other was stronger than ever. God had a plan and His plan was a perfect plan. What a blessing.

Two Years Later

After two years the radiation department would continue to be amazed at Doug's remarkable healing. They began to call him one of their *miracles.* They were astounded until they finally found out we were also using mild hyperbaric oxygen and near infrared light therapy in conjunction with good nutrition. We made these treatments his number one priority as part of his recovery in hopes of guaranteeing long-term healing and preventing the cancer from ever returning.

My hat's off to you Doug, for choosing to live; for allowing me to guide you through your darkest hours, your most painful days and for giving hope a chance. In my eyes you are a rock star. I commend you for focusing on your health and wellness even when you didn't want to; for making the commitment and trusting in me and my belief that oxygen and light therapy would regenerate new blood supply for a more complete healing. Because of this you gained the rejuvenation of your salivary glands and your taste buds and full use of your tongue and jaw without the restriction of scar tissue. Not to mention *you have your brain back!* Thank you for allowing those who love you into your heart and your pain; for cultivating self-respect and a devotion to have a better quality of life filled with happiness. Thank you for loving me and showing up differently in life. Thank you for sharing your story and success with others that are trusting me for guidance, as it gives them hope. You are truly an example to be admired, my love.

In the following chapters I will walk you through the five steps we used to regain Doug's health and get him the healing needed in order to have the quality of life he desired and deserved. Please know that I am not a doctor and do not claim to be a cancer specialist. I am a nurturing, loving, compassionate human who has years of experience helping people heal. These are the therapies and thought processes that helped us through this difficult time and the steps I use to help others.

Step 1: Commit; Show Up, and Learn
Step 2: Dive in and Light Up: Oxygen & Light for Healing
Step 3: Cultivating Healthy Cells
Step 4: Detox and Move
Step 5: Unleash Emotional Baggage

CHAPTER 4

To Heal or Not to Heal

"Believe that there's light at the end of the tunnel.
Believe that you might be that light for someone else."
– Kobi Yamada

Step 1: Commit, Show Up, and Learn

Commitment is the first step toward success of any kind, and your healing isn't any different. Coming out of cancer treatment can be depressing and defeating. Your damage is deep and systemic. Your healing will take time and you have to want it, you have to want to thrive. It is up to you to decide what kind of healing you want; you have to make the commitment. This doesn't mean you are alone—it just means you are the one that needs to be willing to make the lifestyle changes necessary to rebuild your system. You will not heal without making changes. You must change the environment within. Your immune system has been highly compromised. It won't be easy, but now you get to choose what's next. These are my questions for you:

- Do you love yourself enough to do the work?
- Are you going to clean house and get all the dirt and bugs out?
- What kind of cells will you grow? Will they be plump, healthy and energetic? Or will they be mutated, angry, and lazy?
- Will the environment be ripe for more cancer to return?

The choice is yours…

Mary's Story

Commitment looks different during various times of your healing. Because the damage is so devastating and affects your entire body, there will be times when you're barely functioning. Take my client Mary, for example: she is a sweet, 78-year-old woman who had just finished chemotherapy when she came to me. Her daughter was with her because she was so sick that she was unable to drive. As she told me about her chemotherapy journey, I could tell she was an independent type of gal. In the beginning of her treatment she thought, "I can do this, no problem." But each chemo treatment took away more and more of her independence and it took her longer and longer to recover. Her energy was very low, she felt a little dizzy and she was having a tough time getting through the day on her own. She was becoming forgetful, life seemed really foggy and she could not get rid of the nauseated feeling in her stomach. She was also experiencing tingling and shooting pain in her feet, bothering her at night so much that she couldn't sleep.

She explained that her friend had told her how much she loved coming to our office and that hyperbaric oxygen, light and vibration helped her heal after treatment. Mary wasn't quite sure about any of this, as it was so new to her. But she wanted her life back, so she was willing to try anything and the doctors weren't able to help her. They wanted her to take Gabapentin for her feet, but it made her drowsy all day and she really wanted to get back to her gardening—not to mention it didn't really help her pain much. She just didn't want to be on any more drugs.

We talked about the basics: her diet, bowel movements and hydration. She was barely getting any nutrition. Everything she ate was out of a box: cold cereal and pasta, things that were easy for her to make on her own. Her bowel movements reflected the combination of what she was eating and the constipating effects of chemo drugs: They were like hard golf balls that were sometimes painful coming out. She didn't really like drinking water so she would drink juice or sometimes a soda. I made a list of foods to incorporate into her diet and some meal suggestions to make it easier for her. We talked about proper hydration and how it would dramatically change the way she feels and help her to detox the chemicals out of her body. I recommended she talk to her doctor about going in for hydro-colon therapy to help get her bowels moving.

Then I took her and her daughter on a tour of our office and explained how the hyperbaric oxygen and light therapy may help her body to heal itself. I told her about other patients similar to her who had experienced success with increased energy, more brain clarity and better internal function after some of my therapies. We also talked about how the near infrared lights are FDA-approved for increasing circulation and reducing pain and inflammation, so could give her the relief she needed in her feet. It was all a little overwhelming for her, but she was committed to her health and wanted to get back to enjoying life. With the help of her daughter, she jumped in with both feet and made a full commitment to change the way she ate, to start drinking more water, try hydro-colon therapy and to dive right into a series of treatments in the light chamber. When her daughter couldn't drive her she would rely on another family member to bring her. She knew in order to get her healing she had to do something different and ask for help. *She wanted to heal fast and strong.* Over the next couple of months, it was such a joy working with her and watching her come back to life. She is the perfect example of what it means to commit to your health and healing, even if it means learning new stuff about your body after 78 years. You go girl!

Showing Up

Sometimes your loved ones want you to make changes more than you want it yourself, but at the end of the day, it's up to you. They can help you and support you, but you have to be the one who is committed to your journey. Either you're all in or you're wasting time. Being committed isn't limited to one specific action, it is a combination of mental attitude and passion that these actions grow out of. If you are not truly devoted to your health and you really don't care if you heal, you are wasting the time, energy and love of your caregiver or loved one. Be honest with yourself and them, be open-minded and willing to change directions along the journey.

Doug's Decision to Commit

When I was in the role of caregiver and loving wife during my husband's cancer recovery, it broke my heart to see him in pain and helpless. I wanted to help him as much as I possibly could. This was not an easy task for me, as I had also taken a few falls during this time and tore my rotator cuff, split my bicep tendon and damaged my knee. These additional injuries I had endured were just icing on the cake to my other health conditions that had mostly resolved just before Doug's diagnoses. I felt like my life was emotionally and physically spiraling downwards at every turn I made. Even though I had injured myself and was in need of surgery, I felt his needs had to come first. I still wanted to help him. He was tube-fed for seven months and it was very painful for me to feed him. But knowing that he was unable to feed himself, I was committed to waking up at 5 a.m. every morning to prepare his bag with the best food possible for his healing, make sure he had the supplements needed to grow healthy cells and give him meds and water to keep him on schedule. It was a rigid schedule: he had to be fed four times a day. I also made sure that he was at his appointments, that he showered and had clean clothes and I was always thinking ahead. I didn't mind taking care of him and I would do it all over again. I was committed to rebuilding his immune system and healing his wounds.

But after nine months of putting his needs first, it was time for me to get the care I needed. He was now able to start taking over some of his own care. It would be a struggle for many different reasons. He didn't have the same commitment to his health and healing that I did and he didn't have the knowledge or the passion to stay on track. Eating was now his job—it was critical to his survival and quality of life. He had lost his taste buds and most of his salivary glands so eating was no longer enjoyable. He was careless about timing his meals and sometimes even skipped them, so his weight started dropping. Even though he had a written schedule for his medications and supplements, he was not always compliant. Depression set in and all of a sudden he found himself not feeling well. His energy was low and his pain and anxiety increased.

Part of this was because he never had an interest in health and didn't fully understand the value of good nutrition as well as the role it played in his healing. The other part of it was depression and fear; fear of failing and fear of the future. But having been married to him for 15 years, I knew he had never been committed to his health. He took it for granted because he had always been pretty healthy—so he thought. I would support him in a limited way, but I needed to get out of the way so he could choose. He had to get to the point where he really wanted to heal; to dig deep inside and decide to love himself fully, to forgive himself for things in the past and allow himself to be more present in his future. He had to be responsible for the future of his immune system and he could no longer take it for granted. That's when he committed to learn more about health and nutrition, do more exercise and movement to regain function and to love more fully and show up for himself. He just had to decide he was worth it. It was like he threw a switch and a light bulb came on. Once he committed to himself he was able to be a better husband, friend and caregiver to me through my surgeries. It was a beautiful time in our relationship; it was that "perfect gift from God."

I encourage you to make a conscious decision to take responsibility for your future and commit to rebuilding a healthy immune system for a more complete healing and better quality of life.

One Day at a Time

Take your healing journey a day at a time, but keep the bigger picture in your mind. What will you choose? Will it be health and healing or more sickness and pain?

If you aren't sure where to start, here are a few commitments to consider:

- Love yourself.
- Don't be afraid of a misstep.
- Ask for help; stay connected and communicate your needs.
- Have a clear vision of what you want and stay the course.
- Be persistent, steadfast and determined.
- Start with baby steps and commit to small changes.
- Visualize success.
- Don't be afraid to make adjustments along the way.

- If you have a person, be committed to your person as well. Be a team!
- Read, watch and listen to learn.
- Learn to cook.
- Find purpose and passion.
- Keep your eye on the end game.
- Make affirmation cards so you don't sabotage yourself.

You have a clean slate and you have the power within. Will you commit? What do you want your future to be? How will you re-create yourself?

CHAPTER 5

Dive in and Light Up: Healing with Oxygen & Light

"Hope changes everything."
– Unknown

Step 2: Our Primal Nutrients

Through my experience working with clients who are healing from the devastation of traditional cancer treatments, two things stand out: the slow healing and the long-term damage.

Due to a weakened immune system and damaged blood vessels, the healing process can be slow and grueling. Not only is it frustrating and discouraging, but the longer your cells have to struggle, the more scar tissue you'll develop. If you can feed your cells the needed nutrients, you can speed up your healing process for a healthier and more complete healing.

I have had both personal and professional experience healing with and without hyperbaric oxygen and light therapy. I can say without a doubt that I would no longer want to be without either of these healing tools. Everyone's healing experience may be different, but one thing is universal for everyone: Oxygen and light are the primal nutrients for all life. When chemotherapy and radiation suck the life out of you, the next step should be to dive into a hyperbaric oxygen chamber, bathing your cells with light while breathing deeply and let go of the stress. It will bring you back to living your life healthier and stronger!

Oxygen as a Nutrient

Oxygen is the most important key element in life. It's your primary source of energy and the fuel required for your cells to operate properly. We can live several days without water, a few weeks without food, but only a few minutes without oxygen. Oxygen is critical for cell regeneration and is required for any type of healing. Oxygen is necessary for food mobilization and the elimination of toxins and waste. It is mandatory for movement, seeing, eating, sleeping, talking and thinking. Because all the functions in your body are regulated by oxygen, it must be replaced endlessly because your life depends upon it. Without oxygen there would be no life.

What Is Hyperbaric Oxygen Therapy?

Hyperbaric Oxygen Therapy (HBOT) is a way for you to breathe oxygen at pressures greater than at sea level. Under normal circumstances, oxygen is transported throughout the body only by red blood cells. When you're injured, diseased, or even through normal aging, you develop inflammation that causes restrictions in your blood vessels. Your red blood cells are too large to get through the restricted vessel and are no longer able to carry oxygen to the tissue on the other side. That tissue becomes very unhealthy without its steady stream of fresh oxygen. This is when you begin to have pain, tingling, numbness, weakness or total breakdown of tissue. Breathing oxygen under pressure pushes the oxygen through your lungs and dissolves it into your blood plasma and cerebral-spinal fluid. These fluids can now carry oxygen into the starving tissue and begin to reduce inflammation. When inflammation is reduced, blood flow increases the delivery of oxygen into deprived areas and the body can support its own healing process.

Three different types of hyperbaric oxygen chambers and treatment are done at various pressures using various percentages of oxygen. Hospitals use mono chambers that look like glass tubes that are pressurized with 100% oxygen at high pressures. The patient will breathe and bathe in 100% oxygen. There are 15 FDA-approved indications that are covered when having treatment in a hospital setting. This is usually reserved for very sick people or wounds that will not heal. These treatments can be dangerous and toxic to the body if not delivered properly and monitored closely.

There are also multi-place chambers where many people can be treated at the same time. These can be operated at varying pressures but are pressurized with ambient (room) air. The oxygen is delivered to the client through a hood, cannula or mask.

The chambers that we use are mild portable chambers that are pressurized at 4 psi (1.3 ata) with ambient air. There is fresh air flowing through the chamber continually during treatment, but the pressure will stay the same. Our clients breathe concentrated oxygen through a mask or cannula, or can even have the oxygen free flow into the chamber if desired. Many professionals don't believe that these chambers are powerful enough to make changes in the body. Through my personal and professional healing experiences, I beg to differ. I have many stories as well as before and after photos to prove the healing qualities of mild hyperbaric therapy. These chambers are FDA-approved but most of the healing that takes place is not acknowledged by the FDA. We are simply helping the body in its own ability to heal by feeding it a supplement of the very nutrient that keeps us alive and aids our cells in the repair process. It is a supplement of oxygen!

Mild HBOT treatment times range from 60 to 90 minutes and are preferably administered daily, and sometimes twice daily, five days a week. The goal is to keep the levels of oxygen in the bodily fluids higher than normal for a longer period of time. After receiving hyperbaric oxygen therapy, there will be increased oxygen in the plasma for around three hours. If one is using this therapy for healing, it is recommended that you rest and relax during these three hours, allowing oxygen to dissipate into the tissue for healing. If you want to speed up the healing process, a second treatment within four hours is recommended. If you are taking oxygen therapy to increase stamina or endurance, you would spend this time exercising.

It is a simple, safe, non-invasive and painless treatment and, in my opinion, it's the best-kept secret in the medical profession. Who doesn't want to heal faster and more completely? With mild hyperbaric oxygen therapy this is what I have experienced and witnessed over and over again. Myself, my husband and my clients have healed faster, slept better, experienced more energy, are more relaxed and enjoyed an overall feeling of wellness.

Light as a Nutrient

Light is the mother of all life. Simply stated, life on Earth would not be possible without it. Sunlight keeps us warm and keeps the earth habitable. It makes our gardens grow, gives us the colors of the rainbow and we all feel healthier and happier when the sun is out. Light is a necessary supplement for our bodies and can help regulate mood, sleep, energy, healing and even reduce pain and inflammation. I began using LED light therapy as a healing technique over a decade ago, and it has proven to be one of the most important nutrients for energy, pain management, circulation, mood and sleep. We typically don't consider light as a supplement, but that is how I would like you to contemplate it for your health. Think of it as a daily dose of sunshine directed to the areas of the body that need it the most, the areas that have been damaged and need attention, love and care.

What Is Light Therapy?

Light therapy has been used for thousands of years and is being used more and more in mainstream medicine. Different light waves are used for different purposes. We use X-rays to take photos of the inside of our bodies, as well as to kill unwanted cells with X-ray radiation for cancer tumors. Microwaves are used to heat our food and we use the shorter waves for communication such as TV and radio. On the light spectrum, the healthy rays are visible light and infrared light waves. Sometimes they are used as a laser beam of light for pain, an infrared lamp or blanket or as coherent light through Light Emitting Diodes (LED). Infrared light waves increase circulation and manage pain to aid the body in its natural healing process. The most researched light waves for pain are the red and near-infrared for increasing circulation and reducing pain and inflammation and far-infrared for increasing circulation and detoxification.

When working with clients who are suffering with pain, I use LED light therapy devices that are flexible pads that wrap directly around the body against the skin so the body can absorb the light energy. Near-infrared energy releases nitric oxide from hemoglobin and endothelial cells. Nitric oxide is a signaling molecule that relaxes smooth muscle cells found in the arteries, veins and lymph vessels. When these muscles relax, the vessels dilate, thus allowing increased circulation locally. Visualize your veins carrying more blood and oxygen to the injured area for healing.

When placing the light pads directly on the skin, you will feel a gentle warmth from the diodes and it will stimulate a healing response deep inside the body. A light therapy session lasts 20 minutes, after which you can then move the pad to surrounding areas if you wish.

A Match Made in Heaven

You are sick and injured from radiation and chemotherapy. You are in pain, inflamed, have low energy and your blood circulation is compromised. Light and oxygen are the most important primal nutrients for you at this time. Oxygen is critical for your healing and light stimulates circulation to carry oxygen to the damaged areas. Through my experience I have not found a better match than mild hyperbaric oxygen and light therapies administered together as a light chamber: a pressurized chamber that uses both light and oxygen therapies to help a patient to heal.

While in the chamber you will not only increase your oxygen intake and circulation, you will also experience the rest and relaxation needed to heal.

The autonomic nervous system is responsible for regulating the body's unconscious actions. Our nervous system has two modes that we operate in: the sympathetic and the parasympathetic. The sympathetic is the "fight or flight" mode. When we are sick, in pain, stressed and over-tired, that is where we typically live, and it is not supportive to healing. The parasympathetic mode is "rest and digest." We heal when we sleep or when we are able to rest and relax because we are not tensed up. Because light therapy is warm and relaxing and your body is getting the primal nutrients it needs, you are able to rest and relax inside the chamber to support your healing.

How Does It Help Me Heal After Radiation and Chemotherapy?

High doses of radiation are used to destroy cancer cells, but they also kill healthy cells in their path. Chemotherapy does the same thing but in a different way. One or both of these harsh treatments may affect your organ function, create open wounds inside and out, induce muscle stiffness and weakness, as well as damage your blood vessels, glands and bones. Some of these side effects will heal within weeks of radiation or chemotherapy, but some can become devastating long-term problems.

When you went in for your cancer treatment, unquestionably you were focused on killing the cancer so you could live. You really didn't think much about what your life might look like after treatment was over, or years down the road. You took for granted that your body would heal like it always does. You never imagined your body would be so broken from treatment that it wouldn't be able to function the way it used to. You knew that your immune system would be compromised, but it was hard to envision exactly what that meant. Before treatment began you were unable to comprehend the devastating effect these treatments would have on your body. Now your body no longer has heathy oxygen delivery, which is critical to your healing process. You will heal over time, but you want to feel better sooner and now that you are finished with treatment, you want to get back to your life. You are also worried about your cancer coming back in the future. To prevent this from happening you need to change the internal environment inside your body.

Breathing oxygen under pressure combined with light therapy are perfect to assist you in this process. As I learned at a conference from Dr. Zayd Ratansi, together they will help your body to regenerate new blood vessels and carry oxygen to your damaged tissue, increase cellular energy and support your body in speeding up the healing process.

Clinical Healing

When you commit to healing in a light chamber, your body is healing as a whole. This is one of the things I love about hyperbaric oxygen therapy: it doesn't know where the damage is, but the therapy supports every system, every organ and every cell. While you are laying in the chamber breathing concentrated oxygen, bathing in healthy light waves and feeding your plasma its most primal nutrients, your body is healing as a whole. It is healing in ways you will never know. It's magical.

This magic comes with a warning; a warning to do the time necessary for long-term healing. It is not unusual that after a short period of treatment you will feel so good you will want to go live your life and not make time for your continued program. But as you probably know, after having radiation or chemotherapy your body is damaged on many different levels. Some of the areas you will find yourself healing very quickly, other areas may take time because you need to re-establish new blood vessels, such as areas with bone or organ necrosis or damaged glands. It takes time to grow new blood vessels. As I tell my clients, you don't grow a garden overnight, so don't expect to grow a new body overnight. A good example of this is Doug's salivary glands and taste buds. It wasn't until about 20 months into his healing that his salivary glands started producing so much saliva that he began drooling in bed without needing to have some kind of added moisture in his mouth through the night. He also no longer had to drink water with every bite of food. This told us that he developed new blood flow to those glands and he now has the long-term healing he wanted so much.

My wish for you is to have a more complete healing and to feel better than you did before cancer invaded your life. Hyperbaric oxygen and light therapy can help you in that process. Give it a chance! Make the commitment!

CHAPTER 6

Cultivating Healthy Cells

"Every time you eat or drink something, you are either feeding disease or fighting it."
– Heather Morgan

Step 3: Hydrate and Eat the Rainbow

We live in a culture of eating fast food without even thinking about the long-term effects it will have on our health. Our bodies are temples and our most important tools for living a productive and happy life, yet we tend to abuse them daily by not really thinking about what's best for our organs, muscles, tissues, blood and brain. If we plant a garden or a tree in our yard, we would think about the health of the soil that feeds the roots, how much sun it will receive and how much water it will need. Our bodies are no different than the plants in our yard, yet many of us go about our day not giving a thought to how much nutrition is in our food, how much water we should drink or the exercise and movement we need to strengthen our muscles and tissues. We go obliviously throughout our day and are surprised when disease invades our lives.

A healthy lifestyle that cultivates habits of eating real food and thinking about nutrition and hydration is important. For a cancer patient who has just gone through conventional radiation and chemotherapy, it is crucial. These harsh cancer treatments have destroyed your immune system. Your immune system is strengthened and rejuvenated by what you feed your cells and you will not be able to heal if you are consuming the same food that made you sick. You must change the environment within.

Nutrition is a process in which food is taken in by the body for growth, energy production and rejuvenation of damaged cells. Eating the right kind of food will help you to feel better and stronger and heal faster. It is important to learn about acidic versus alkaline foods so you can make better choices and balance your body's pH levels. All of us have cancer cells in our bodies, and it is the job of the immune system to keep those cancer cells in check. The goal should be to cultivate more healthy cells than cancer cells. Cancer cells rely on the first part of the energy production process which is dependent on glucose (sugar). If you want to stay healthy, I highly recommend that you eliminate sugar from your diet once you have gone through cancer treatment.

When my husband was dying of cancer and had a feeding tube that went directly into his stomach, he had to be feed a tube feeding formula. I was appalled when I read the ingredients of the formula that they gave him. On the front of the container it said in bold print: vanilla, artificially flavoured. If it's fed via a feeding tube, why would you need it to be flavored? Along with that, here are the top three ingredients of that formula:

- Water
- Maltodextrin (a polysaccharide that is used as a food additive. It is commonly used for the production of soft drinks and candy. It can also be found as an ingredient in a variety of other processed foods.)
- Sugar

Water, sugar, and a bunch of chemicals that mimic vitamins. This man is dying of cancer and they give him sugar! All I could think about was that he would never heal if this was all he had as "nourishment" for his sick body. After a lot of research and talking to the nutritional therapist at the hospital, I found a "whole food" tube feeding formula that would give my husband the nutrition he needed to give him a balanced diet and protect his healthy cells. This formula called "Liquid Hope" gave him a good foundation to restore his immune system and rebuild his damaged tissue.

When we began weaning Doug off of the feeding tube, the goal was for him to maintain his weight by only being fed by mouth. He would need to maintain his weight for one month without using the feed tube before they would remove it. Since he was re-learning how to eat, we needed to give him well balanced high density, high quality, rich in nutrient shakes. We could make our own but because I was trying to get back to work I began looking for something to replace the "Liquid Hope". In my research I found "Komplete" nutritional shakes made by Kate Farms. These meal replacement shakes are organic, plant-based protein and are free from dairy, gluten, soy and corn. I recommend you read the story about this company, it is a sweet story and an amazing product. Having these shakes in the refrigerator gave Doug some independence, the nutrition he needed and me some peace of mind.

It is also important to consider supplementing your diet with vitamins and minerals. Everyone's needs are different, so it's best to work with a good nutritional therapist or naturopathic doctor to help guide you through your healing journey. There are many more nutritional recommendations I have for changing the environment within, which I have listed below. Educate yourself!

Nutritional recommendations for a stronger immune system

- Eliminate all processed sugars before anything else
- Eliminate processed foods altogether—focus on eating the rainbow
- Juicing: Raw, cold-pressed juice absorbs directly into the blood stream
- Probiotics to replenish healthy gut flora
- Bone broth to heal the lining of the gut
- Infusions of vitamin C. (Consult with your naturopath)
- Aloe vera supplements
- Vitamins B and D, and SUNSHINE!
- Chia seeds and fiber to support toxin removal from the bowels
- High quality fish oil
- Mushroom extracts
- Melatonin
- Turmeric
- Garlic
- Medicinal marijuana tinctures
- Coconut water—hydrating and full of electrolytes

Resources and diet references

- The Gerson Therapy
- Ketogenic Diet
- Forks Over Knives
- Chrisbeatcancer.com

Essential Oils

Incorporating high quality, food-grade essential oils into your routine is a must. I recommend looking into their therapeutic healing properties, especially for frankincense in particular. It's used most commonly for supporting those battling cancer because it has demonstrated its powerful healing capabilities. The oil of frankincense has been used for thousands of years to quell disease-causing inflammation, strengthen immune defenses and prevent high-risk infections. It can be used both topically and orally.

Our Body of Water

Most of the human body is made up of water and water is the primary building block of our cells. Chemotherapy, radiation, opiates and all other medications used during cancer treatment are dehydrating. They suck the water right out of you. Water regulates our internal body temperature and radiation burns your body and therefore raises your internal temperatures. It's like tiny little campfires raging throughout your system, depleting your cells of their water reserves. Drinking lots of water is critical to help in cooling your body and replenishing the reserves used up by these treatments. Water is also crucial in helping your body to produce saliva, which is the beginning of your digestive process. One of the most concerning side effects of traditional cancer treatment is constipation. Well, go figure! Consider it a domino effect on the body. Toxin overload, dehydration, constipation, followed by nausea and sluggishness. If you are not eliminating properly, your nausea will be harder to manage. Water is essential to flush waste and toxins out of the body through sweat, urination and bowel movements. So drink up and remember to choose only the purest, most alkaline water you can find. Avoid plastic water bottles, tap water and flavored water as these are toxic and hard on the body, especially when you're cleaning house and working to rejuvenate your body for a brighter and healthier tomorrow!

CHAPTER 7

Clean the Tank and Make Waves

"Take care of your body, it is the only place you have to live in."
— Jim Rohn

Step 4: Detox and Move

Detoxification needs to be an important part of your program. You don't have to be a rocket scientist to know that chemotherapy and radiation are extremely toxic. Many of the negative affects you may have from your treatment are from the toxic overload.

This analogy may seem off the wall, but it helps to have a visual. I love turtles and for years our only pets were aquatic turtles. We have three of them and the largest one is the size of a dinner plate. They all live in an 80-gallon tank. They eat a variety of foods, but their all-time favorite is goldfish. They can demolish 50 fish in a matter of minutes and the tank will look like a killing field. Over the following few days the filter will clean up the mess and the water will be clean again. However, out of sight is a disgusting filter that needs to be cleaned. If we don't clean the filter soon thereafter, the tank will become murky and unhealthy for the turtles and the water will stop flowing through the filter.

Your body is like the turtle tank. You overload it with toxins from the food you eat, chemicals in the environment, air you breath and even emotional baggage. There's a good chance that toxins played a role in the growth of your cancer. Now, to add insult to injury, your system is overburdened with not only the chemo, radiation and drugs, but also with the toxic waste of your body breaking down the tumor and dead tissue. You have a built-in filter system that works really well for you—until it is overloaded. How do you know when it's overloaded? When you have symptoms.

Pay special attention to what your body is telling you, then ask the questions: Are you eliminating properly? How are your bowels and urination working? Do you have skin issues or a cough? Do you have headaches or confusion? Could this be a manifestation of toxic overload?

Your filtration system is made up of many organs in your body: your liver, kidneys, intestines, skin, respiratory tract and lymph system all work together to constantly filter toxins internally. You then have to get those toxins out of your body. The main exit organs are your bowels, urinary tract, lungs and skin. There are many ways to assist your organs in this ongoing, everyday task. I highly recommend a cleanse, not a fast. Doing intermittent fasting is fine—especially overnight, but not fasting for days. To cleanse and have your body respond well, your organs need support. I suggest that you work with a professional for guidance when choosing the right cleanse for you, but please don't starve yourself.

Oxygen Therapy for Detox

Breathing increased oxygen under pressure dissolves oxygen into the cerebral fluids, and allows for more absorption. It can reduce the time that toxic substances remain in the brain. When oxygen in the brain is increased through the cerebral fluids, it supplies the cells with the nutrients they need to heal and release the toxic overload.

When Trina came in to see me she had what they call "chemo brain" and was addicted to opiates because of her post-surgical pain. She desperately wanted to get back to living life and she felt like she was in a dark cave. She was afraid of what would happen if she stopped taking her opiates, she was scared about withdrawal symptoms and worried about how much pain she would feel. She started doing daily doubles in the hyperbaric oxygen chamber. After two sessions she felt lifted out of her depression and within fifteen sessions she was a changed woman. There was not a day where she had withdrawal symptoms from her opiates, she was thinking more clearly, she was sleeping through the night and her pain was practically nonexistent. It is such a natural process for the body to move through, it's a beautiful thing to see someone come out of such a dark place. I highly recommend using the far-infrared Sauna after your oxygen dives for even better detoxification.

Far-Infrared Sauna

Sitting in a sauna is a great way to sweat toxins out of the body. All saunas are great, but specifically far-infrared saunas are wonderful for cancer survivors. Regular wet saunas heat you from the outside-in; infrared saunas heat you from the inside-out. They are heated by carbon panels that emit far-infrared light waves which penetrate deep into the body, heating you from the inside. These light waves are present in the natural light spectrum and are created by our sun, other stars and other warm objects like light bulbs, and are very effective for breaking up toxins and fat cells and sweating them out via the skin. Far-infrared saunas allow you to receive more benefit at lower temperatures, making it easier to stay in for longer periods of time.

Bio Mat technology is another beneficial way to detoxify with far-infrared light waves. This technology is delivered through a flexible pad made to fit the bed (with different size options) and radiates far-infrared heat through amethyst crystals. This is particularly helpful when one can't handle the heat, sit up for extended periods of time or if therapy is needed in bed.

Please note that, during detoxification, accumulated toxins are released from cells and organs. The movement of these toxins through the body may produce sensations that are uncomfortable or might feel as though you're getting sick. This is what we call a "healing crisis": the body is going through a healing process, so just take it slow, get plenty of rest and drink lots of water. These symptoms should subside within a few hours.

Coffee Enemas and Colonics

If you have never heard of hydro-colon therapy or coffee enemas, I highly recommend you try both. It is not the most fun therapy, but they work well together and your body will love you for it. As you know by now, the toxic overload from your treatments have wreaked havoc on your intestinal tract and you are probably experiencing constipation. If you had chronic bowel problems before your cancer, you may not understand what normal bowel movements should be like. Most people don't like to talk about their bowels, but I can't stress enough how important they are in giving us messages about our general health. In a perfect world, you would have 2-4 bowel movements a day that are perfectly formed like a banana and that look and feel complete. If you are pooping golf balls that are hard to push out once a day, you are constipated—and this is not a healthy state. Colon therapy and coffee enemas assist in removing stuck toxic waste and parasites from the gut. They help stimulate your liver to support detoxification, as well as rebalance gut flora and promote healing. I always recommend checking in with your doctor or healthcare provider before starting any new therapy. If your car needed an oil and filter change, you would not hesitate to take care of it. Why wouldn't you take care of your body in the same way?

Coffee enemas are something you do in the comfort of your home using a special coffee enema kit and organic light roast ground coffee boiled in purified water. The goal is to fill your colon with the coffee and hold it for 15-20 minutes before releasing it. I encourage you to find videos on YouTube about "how to do a coffee enema"—there are lots of them.

When coffee is used as an enema, it stimulates the production of glutathione by the liver. Glutathione is a powerful antioxidant and cellular protector; it also stimulates the liver to remove toxic waste out of our cells. Studies show that green coffee beans can boost this production in the liver. The coffee enema has powerful effects because the enzymes of the digestive tract don't interact with the nutrient before they reach the liver.

There are many different types of enema kits. My favorite is from the Gerson Institute. You can order it on Gerson.org and it comes with a package of organic green coffee. Be easy on yourself when learning how to do coffee enemas, as practice makes perfect and this can be a very powerful tool in your healing and keeping your "tank" clean.

Hydro-colon therapy is a process where your colon is filled with purified water through the rectum to hydrate and assist you in cleansing stuck waste out of the colon. This is done in a professional setting with special equipment to make the process comfortable and safe. If you are having chronic constipation, it is best to schedule a series of appointments close together to get the best outcome. It is not the most enjoyable process, but most people will feel so much better afterwards and your colon will work more efficiently. Although coffee enemas are usually done at home, some hydro-colon therapists are willing to assist you with a coffee enema after your colonics if you bring the coffee in with you. Happy cleansing!

Green Clay Masks

Another powerful tool to assist your body in removing toxins is green clay masks. This is a very simple technique that is used to pull toxins out of the skin. You can purchase organic green clay on Amazon or from your local naturopath. Just mix organic green clay with organic castor oil, then apply it directly on the skin and leave for one to two hours. This can be especially powerful in areas where you have been radiated. Beginning these treatments when radiation therapy starts, before the skin is broken down, may eliminate the possibility of external burning. I did a clay mask on Doug over his neck and face two to three times a week when he was beginning the first week of radiation. At the end of treatment, he was the only one walking around without a severe sunburn. Nurse Angela could not believe how beautiful and healthy the skin on his neck and face was. It takes some extra time and attention, but it is so worth it when you see how badly others can be burned by radiation. Remember, the skin is one of your major exit organs to rid toxins from the body. Green clay masks can assist this process and leave you with healthier skin.

Castor Oil Packs

The history of using castor oil for health goes back thousands of years. It has many uses, but is most famous for being used as a strong laxative when used internally. There are several ways to use castor oil topically as well. You can simply rub it onto areas of your body to reduce pain and inflammation, or you can apply a castor oil pack for a more systemic application. When placed over the abdomen or the lower back (for kidneys), it is extremely useful to help with detoxification, reducing inflammation and stimulating lymphatic circulation. You can use castor oil packs through your treatments to assist in daily detoxification to support your body. Castor oil packs are made with three layers of organic flannel soaked with organic castor oil and are best applied with a heat pack protected with plastic. When doing a castor oil pack, it is best done at bedtime or when you are able to lay down and rest for 45 to 60 minutes. Coming out of chemo and radiation can feel like coming home from battle—castor oil packs are a soothing and easy way to help your body recover.

Mud Baths

One of my personal favorite therapies for detoxification is a hypothermia mud bath. This therapy is best used after treatment is completed. If you are fighting infection, a cold, have increased pain, or need to get an overnight response from your body, the mud bath should be your choice. However, you should not use this therapy if you have open wounds and I advise checking with your doctor before you try it.

It looks very similar to taking a bath in coffee. Before getting in the tub, prepare your bed with layers of towels to lay on and a towel and several blankets to cover you. The goal is to have your bath water as hot as possible, add the bottle of Naked Mud, stir it up and soak for 15-20 minutes. When you are ready to get out, pat yourself dry and get to your bed as quickly as you can while trying not to lose too much heat. Cover yourself up to your neck, arms and all and sweat for 30 minutes. It is best to do before bed and wake up a changed person!

Movement

Exercise creates waves in the body to assist our internal filtration system to move toxins out and keep our muscles strong and healthy. Try to exercise as much as possible during treatment and recovery, as it is critical to your healing. The more you can keep moving and exercising, the less function you will lose and the better you will feel. When you are sick, it's easy to fall into a depressed state and become sedentary, but do your best to avoid this pitfall. Unless you have a lot of pain or are unable to move, it is smart to have a regular exercise routine, even if it's just walking and using a few free weights. Here are some ways that regular exercise may help you during and after treatment:

- Keep muscles from wasting away
- Bring oxygen to your cells
- Lower the occurrence of anxiety and depression
- Combat fatigue
- Lessen nausea
- Lower the risk for blood clots

- Better balance which lowers your risk of falls
- Improve self-esteem
- Help rebuild immune system

Go for walks outside in the sunshine as much as you can, your body needs the natural light to boost your vitamin D. "From a scientific point of view, vitamin D reduces the risk of developing many types of cancer and increases survival once cancer reaches the detectable stage." (Mercola, 2009). Between getting out in the sunshine and incorporating movement into your daily routine, you are increasing your chances of a better outcome in recovery. If you are very sick or in pain, do your best to get up and move throughout the house. Your caregiver can help you put together a small daily routine with simple exercises like leg lifts and moving your arms above your head even if you don't have any weights. You may even want to look for a personal trainer that can come into the home and work with you. Even if you feel sick, sitting around without movement will not serve you well and may give you additional problems.

Doug's Lack of Movement

Doug was in bed or on the couch for two months, only going to and from the hospital for his treatments. As I shared with you early on, his blood pressure would drop considerably from lying, to sitting, to standing—it's a condition called orthostatic hypotension. He suffered through many fainting spells, falls and rounds of tests to ultimately find out that a big part of it was because he had been sedentary for too long. If he had had a simple exercise program, it could have saved him from additional side effects. What a lesson this was!

Whole Body Vibration

If you have been cleared by your doctor, Whole Body Vibration may be a good option for your exercise routine, and one that I have been using at my healing center with my clients. Simply defined, Whole Body Vibration is stimulus motion delivered to the body through a mechanical platform. These movements engage your muscle fibers. Thousands of involuntary muscle contractions are triggered throughout your body, naturally stimulating every cell, including your muscles, bone and soft tissue. By way of movement at the cellular level, increasing circulation and stimulating your lymphatic system you are strengthening your body's natural defenses and overall energy. There are many different vibration platforms available; some just have vibration and others have vibration and oscillation, which mimics walking. I recommend you seek guidance from a professional to design a vibration plan specific to you. The benefits may include increased muscle strength, circulation and bone density; reduced pain; and an improvement in balance and coordination.

Jolene and Her Neuropathy

When I started working with Jolene, she was suffering with neuropathy in her feet caused by chemotherapy. Neuropathy is the damage and death of nerve fibers that can be caused by diabetes, chemotherapy, trauma, pharmaceuticals and more. It can be extremely painful and debilitating, ultimately leading to the dying of limbs and amputation in extreme cases or if left untreated. Jolene was struggling so much that she was unable to exercise on her own. We had her coming in for daily infrared light therapy sessions followed by low intensity vibration. Within weeks her neuropathy was nearly gone, she was sleeping through the night and she was able to walk her dog again. It was a beautiful thing for us to witness such a drastic and positive change in her quality of life by incorporating just a few very simple modalities into her routine!

CHAPTER 8

Unleash Emotional Garbage

"All you need is love."
– John Lennon

Step 5: Let Go and Live

Trapped emotions can make us sick. For so many years this area of knowledge has been overlooked and unappreciated. It's just now finally starting to be recognized by practitioners and healers in the industry. Emotions can be harbored in areas of our bodies for years, eventually leading to physical degenerative diseases that show up in many different forms. Releasing these emotions can set us free and help us heal. Learning the tools and seeking out professional help would be my first recommendation for anyone on their healing journey. It's not something we generally think about when we consider recovery, but it is extremely important.

When you were diagnosed with cancer, you probably wondered how you got it. Was it because of your unhealthy diet or lifestyle? Was it due to your toxic environment at work? Did genetics play a role? But rarely will somebody diagnosed with cancer ask themselves, "What toxic emotion am I harboring that could have played a role?" In most cases, this is always a factor involved in the onset of this awful disease. (E-Motion: The Movie, 2014).

Emotions are very powerful and we all have emotional baggage that gets in the way of living life and having healthy relationships with ourselves and others. Each emotion has its own vibrational frequency and, when we have intense emotional experiences, those vibrations can become like a trapped ball of energy that we don't realize is there. They can cause disruptions in our overall energy system and eventually cause physical disease. Even the American Medical Association now recognizes that emotions have a direct connection to our health. Emotions that grow out of a chronic state of stress play a major factor in 90% of all health problems.

As you go through the healing process, you know exactly where you need physical healing, but it's the emotional scars that are not visible and may hinder your healing process. Sometimes the people around us can see what is hindering us more than we can. Don't be afraid to ask your loved ones or your closest friends to have an honest conversation about what they see in you emotionally. Or consider working with an emotional healing professional. While you are moving through your journey, you may feel impending failure and fear of the future. This is normal, but if you allow it to control your thoughts through anxiety and stress, you are feeding the devil.

There are many techniques to help you uncover trapped emotions and release them to regain balance and harmony for a more complete healing and a fuller life. Here are a few that you may want to research:

- Emotional Freedom Technique (EFT)
- Freedom Release Technique (FreedomRT)
- The Emotion Code
- Access Consciousness
- Body Talk
- The Sedona Method

"Healing doesn't mean the damage never existed. It means the damage no longer controls our lives."
— Akshay Dubey

Law of Attraction

Maybe you have heard about "The Secret" or the "Law of Attraction" series. The basic premise of the Law of Attraction is simply "what you think about, comes about." You have the ability to deliberately create your life the way you want and let go of negative thoughts by replacing them with positive ones that serve you better. I have found this law to be very effective in my own life. It seems farfetched to some, but I have also seen many of my clients either succeed or struggle through their healing journey because of techniques like these. Our thoughts and words are very powerful and can affect the way we feel about ourselves and how it may affect our healing. What we think about, comes about. How many times have you been talking about someone or thinking about them and out of the blue they call you? You have the power to change your thoughts and actions to change your outcome. You have the power to deliberately create your life moving forward. You create your own reality through thoughts, feelings and vibrational energy.

Rob with Intestinal Pain

Rob was a client who came in with severe intestinal pain. He had been to many different doctors and gone through several series of tests that showed no physical damage, disease or tumors. It was a mystery, but nonetheless he was suffering with a great deal of pain. He began coming in for hyperbaric oxygen and light therapy in efforts to reduce his pain. As I got to know him better, it became clear that he had an incredible amount of anger built up towards his ex-wife, as well as anger and resentment from years of abuse from his father. He had negative thoughts running through his mind that would spill over into his conversations. It was obvious to me that these reoccurring negative emotional thoughts and words were causing him a great deal of pain. At his next appointment I planned an exercise that would attempt to turn his negative thoughts and words into positive affirmations. I wanted to see if his emotions were the cause of his pain.

I had him write down ten negative thoughts that played over and over again in his mind. We then took each negative thought and flipped them into positive sentences.

Example:

Negative thought: I am a horrible husband and no woman will ever want me.

Positive Affirmations:

1. I am a loving, caring person looking for the perfect partner.
2. I love myself fully and forgive myself for past mistakes.

Then I had him write the positive sentences on 3 x 5 colored cards and instructed him to keep them close and use them when the negative thoughts came to mind. His homework for the next week was to repeat them in the following ways daily:

- Read them silently
- Read them out loud in a normal voice
- Read them while looking in the mirror
- Say them in a very loud voice when no one is around
- Say them again in a loud voice while holding his hand on his cheek so he could feel the vibration of each word

Within a week, his pain was gone. He was so surprised that he had carried around those negative emotions for so many years and made himself sick. He had wasted hundreds of dollars and countless hours trying to figure out what was wrong with him, when all he needed to do was change his thoughts, words and energy into love and forgiveness toward himself.

The best way to move yourself out of misery is to live in a constant state of love and gratitude. Make a list of all the things you are grateful for and keep it handy. Read them to yourself at least once a day, saying them out loud. I encourage you to always begin with, "I am so grateful for who I am, I am a…" so you remember to love yourself. If we don't love ourselves, we can never truly love others.

Replacing Anger with Love

When Doug was near death, overdosed on opiates and waiting for his feeding tube to be placed, I was so angry at him for the position he had put our family in with his health. As I mentioned, when all of this started we were not in a good place in our marriage. But I knew it would not serve either of us if I continued to hold on to the anger and resentment. I needed to do something to help both of us feel loved, so I picked up a box of little pop-open cards that each had sayings of love inside. Every morning and night, I would open a new card and read it to him. He was so sedated he was not really hearing me, but I knew he would get the message and feel the love. Vibrational energy is powerful in times like this! And what was most important was that *I* was getting the message, as all I could do at that moment was love him. By raising my vibrational frequency through love and gratitude, I was also raising his. It was God's plan.

Have Faith in the Lord

If there is ever a time when you rely on your faith, it's in a time of crisis. I believe this is God's way of getting our attention. It was helpful to us to have our daily prayer book to lift us up and help us remember who is in control. Between the little love cards and the daily prayers, it gave both of us comfort. Rely on your spiritual faith, whatever it may be, to give thanks for each and every day. Have an attitude of gratitude for everything, big and small, and all of those around you. Unleash those trapped emotions and set them free!

"The soul always knows what to do to heal itself. The challenge is to silence the mind."
– Caroline Myss

CHAPTER 9

Thrive in Your World After Breathing in Ours

Stories of Healing with Oxygen and Light

Through my personal and professional experiences of helping others use mild hyperbaric oxygen therapy for pain and healing, I am on a mission to help others understand its power and simplicity. Although the following stories are not all related to cancer, I felt strongly about sharing a variety of stories to help you better understand the power of these primal nutrients and to know this is a therapy available to you and your loved ones. As I watch the changes in my clients after a few sessions of breathing oxygen under pressure and soaking up the waves of light, it has made me realize how we are all deficient in these much-needed nutrients. I welcome you into the stories of others who thrive in their world after breathing in ours.

Breast Cancer Recovery

When Patty came into my office, she had recently finished radiation therapy for breast cancer. She was experiencing pain, reduced movement of her arm and the tissue where she had been radiated was red and sore. She also had concerns about damage to her lungs and the possibility of permanent scarring. She committed herself to daily one-hour hyperbaric oxygen sessions for 20 days. Within a week, her pain was gone and she was able to move her arm and shoulder more freely. The tissue on her breast had noticeably healed and the soreness was drastically reduced. To her surprise, she also felt a huge lift in her energy and was feeling more like herself. By the time she finished her last session, she was feeling nearly back to normal. When she went in for her six-month check-up, her doctor was impressed and surprised that her radiated breast tissue was soft and supple instead of the typical radiated tissue being fibrotic and hard. He wanted to know what she did that was different. She also shared with me that a friend of hers went through breast cancer at the same time as she did, and her friend not only had hard scar tissue and flexibility problems, but was now facing a recurrence of cancer.

Neuropathy from Chemotherapy

It broke my heart when Sally came to see me. As she shuffled across the room, I could see that she was in so much pain. She told me about her journey with breast cancer and that she had chemotherapy that ended nine months ago. She was so happy to be in remission, but she had this burning sensation and tingling in her hands and feet that sometimes felt like shooting electrical pain. It would keep her up at night, and she was beginning to lose feeling in two of her toes. This was a side effect of the chemotherapy and the doctors told her there was nothing she could do for it. They told her she was lucky they saved her life but she would have to be on Gabapentin the rest of her life. She did not like taking it and was looking for other options. Her friend had neuropathy up to her knees and had gotten the feeling back all the way to her feet with light therapy, so Sally figured it was worth a try.

She started coming in for daily sessions in the hyperbaric light chamber and she noticed a considerable difference within the first few sessions. She was able to sleep through the night and her hands and feet were not as agitated and burning. By her 25th session she was almost back to normal, she had feeling back in her toes and her hands no longer had any problems. She also noticed that her hair had grown in thicker and her hairdresser noticed too! Sally was grateful for her healing and she wanted to continue treatment at home. She bought herself a set of lights for healing and prevention. Now she can share them with her entire family!

Colorectal Cancer

Jen had just started her radiation and chemo treatments for stage III colorectal cancer when she found my office. She was a retired nurse and knew that she was going to sustain severe damage from her treatments and was looking for alternative care. She was a little skeptical, but after hearing the story about my husband's throat cancer and successful healing through hyperbaric oxygen therapy, she was willing to give it a chance. She began coming in during her treatment and felt like it helped her with her energy and pain. But it was really at the post-treatment return visit to her doctor's office that she knew something remarkable had happened. Her doctor told her she had had the most severe reactions to her chemo and radiation, yet the quickest healing they had seen. They invited her to speak at an upcoming patient event to talk about what alternative treatments she used to help her heal. A few days later she walked in and brought tears to my eyes and warmed my heart when she said, "I want you to know that I would do it all over again; not only for the quick healing I have received but the love, care and support you and your staff have given me. You have truly had my back around every turn." Wow, how sweet. That is why I do the work I do, to serve people like her.

Total Knee Replacement

Several months before Doug was diagnosed, I had taken two falls onto concrete floors and shredded the meniscus in my left knee. After caring for my husband through his cancer, it was now my turn for repair as I needed a total knee replacement. Now that I had more experience using the light chamber to accelerate healing, I was excited to see how quickly I would heal.

The day after surgery, I began my daily HBOT sessions. This was all new to me and knee replacement is a *big* deal, so I decided to take the Hydrocodone until I no longer needed it. As the days went on, my pain became more and more excruciating. After a week I called the doctor's office and told them I felt like the Hydrocodone was not working for me, so maybe we should try a different medication. They gave me a prescription for Dilaudid. After two days on Dilaudid, my pain was unbearable and my knee was so red and inflamed it looked infected. After the surgeon examined me, they put me on Morphine for longer-acting pain relief. They really could not do anything else without opening me up, so I figured it was worth a shot.

It took me less than 24 hours on the Morphine to know something was seriously wrong and I needed a change. I am very sensitive to drugs and here I was taking two highly addictive pain medications and I was not feeling drugged, nor was I getting relief. I thought that maybe the drugs were getting in the way of the oxygen's ability to work and maybe the oxygen was metabolizing the drugs right out of my system. It was 11:30 at night, and I made the decision to go off all drugs and get in the chamber. I knew that five hours of chamber time substantially reduces inflammation, which would then reduce the pain. I desperately needed a change, so I went to sleep in the chamber for six hours. When I got out the next morning my pain had gone down and my knee was pink instead of bright red. I would go on to do five more hours that day. When I woke up the next morning, I could hardly believe it. My pain had gone from a 10+ to a 2 on the pain scale in 36 hours' time using oxygen and lights alone. No Meds! My surgeon was perplexed at the speed of my healing and released me after two and a half months. I had full range of motion and hyperextension. This experience taught me some very valuable lessons:

- Prescription medication can get in the way of our body's natural healing process
- HBOT is an amazing detoxification technique
- HBOT can be used as a supportive tool for opiate withdrawal
- How quickly tissue responds when given time, oxygen and light
- Please note: This is not our typical protocol, but nonetheless I had no side effects from the extended time spent in the chamber.

Opiate Addiction from Migraines

I will never forget the anxiety and fear I saw in Katie's face when she came into my office and told me she was addicted to opiates and her doctor would no longer prescribe her pain medication. She was an upstanding business owner in our area who had suffered with migraines since she was 12 years old. Over the years she tried many different medications, but it was the Vicodin that helped get her through the day. Not really thinking about the long-term effects on her health, Katie continued to take 3-5 Vicodins a day for over two years and now she was addicted. She was lost; what was she going to do? Within 24 hours she would have a migraine and nothing to help her. Not only was she afraid of the extreme pain, but also the frightful withdrawal symptoms coming off the opiates.

Katie's first treatment was that afternoon and again late that night. It was important to support her body while coming off the opiates and hopefully use the oxygen as pain relief from her migraine. The next morning she popped in at 7 a.m. with a huge grin on her face and said, "This is the first time I woke up without a migraine in 25 years! I slept so well, I feel great, and have so much more clarity." I was so very happy for her, having suffered with migraines for 30 years myself (before HBOT). I knew how amazing it felt to wake up feeling good after years of suffering. Over the next week she was coming in for two sessions a day. Katie was able to get off her opiates with no with drawl symptoms and did not have a migraine that week. She continued to come in daily for 40 sessions until she bought her own chamber and lights to have at home. Katie knew that the best medicine for her was oxygen and light!

Robin's Traumatic Brain Injury and Concussion

The first day Robin walked in the door of my office, I was concerned as to how much we would be able to help her. She had been in two car accidents within about four months' time, from which she experienced a severe traumatic brain injury as well as other physical damage. As she opened her mouth I could tell it was very difficult for her to get words out. Her walk was a little lopsided and with each step you wanted to hang onto her because she looked like she was going to fall over. She was as sweet as can be and cute as a button with her long curly hair down to her waist. This is her story in her words:

Brain Injury:

"Mental confusion, memory problems, poor concentration, difficulty speaking and understanding, difficulty recognizing common things, difficulty with facial recognition, tinnitus, sensitivity to light and sound, diminished smell and taste, body spasms, vertigo and balance issues, nausea, cachexia, insomnia, fatigue, inappropriate laughing and crying, apathy, impulsivity, lack of restraint, anxiety, irritability, anger, and aggression.

Damage to my peripheral vision and what my medical team believes to be post-traumatic seizures (temporal lobe epilepsy— ecstatic seizures) but there has been suspicion of Transient Ischemic Attacks (TIA or mini strokes). Further diagnostics would be required to appropriately diagnose. Phantom smells (auras of something burning), moments of euphoria followed by confusion and fatigue."

Areas of chronic pain:

"Headaches and migraines, neck, back, right hip and thigh, left side of face/jaw, left hand, wrist, knee, and all of my fingers specifically but my limited understanding is that central pain syndrome sends faulty pain signals to different and sometimes multiple areas of my body at random. So one moment I may feel like freezing water is dripping on me somewhere, and the next I may feel like my heels have been crushed or the skin stripped from my thigh or all of the above plus some. Hyperalgesia, myofascial pain syndrome, dystonia in left wrist."

Changes since HBOT & Light Therapy:

"Increased appetite, improved sleep, flexibility/fluidity in left hand and wrist, better circulation, increased energy and attention to detail for things like personal grooming. Also, I recently noticed less bruising so maybe that means better balance and awareness of surroundings. Less pain in my fingers, some decrease in sensitivity or maybe an increase in tolerance to touch, decrease in both face and body spasms, smell and taste seems to be returning sporadically, and my moments of clarity with both vision and cognitive functioning seem to be extending. I've been thinking a lot about changes in my mood, too. I believed from the start that I had been misdiagnosed with depression and from a more informed place, understand now that I was instead experiencing apathy. With the energy I have recovered from HBOT, I feel enthusiastic about my future again. My anxiety is decreasing and I am able to take so much more in stride, which I think has allowed me to find my words better and improved my speech. This has changed so much because I have since been able to clearly communicate what I am experiencing to the rest of my medical team, and I am now receiving the help I need. Before HBOT, my fears and anxiety ate up the entirety of my appointments and I was prescribed psychotherapy, anti-anxiety, and depression medications instead of having the underlying issues addressed.

I forgot to mention something pretty exciting: I think my recovery time following seizures is shortening. I still feel like I could sleep forever afterward, but it's like clarity comes back much quicker now and it's not so frustrating to get my words out after. I am so very grateful for Edna and her staff at In Light Hyperbarics for standing by me. I feel so blessed to have had the opportunity to have these treatments and hope this brings awareness to others suffering with pain and brain trauma."

Annetta, Retired Nurse and Caregiver—Her story in her words

"I discovered that caring for a 15-year-old granddaughter in crisis, caring for an elderly mother living in my home, entering retirement and selling a home to build another, left me feeling overwhelmed, depressed and stressed.

As a nurse I had unfortunately had a couple of back injuries. I sought help from a chiropractor and was able to maintain a certain degree of improvement, but always needed frequent visits. The years of nursing in difficult environments had also taken a toll and I felt I didn't handle stress well anymore. I wanted and needed change and was ready immediately to try hyperbaric oxygen treatments.

The benefits for me include: a major decrease in inflammation, stabilization of my back pain which has meant fewer trips to a chiropractor and improvement in mental health and feeling like the chamber acts as an antidepressant. My stomach pain also improved dramatically. I noticed a little improvement daily, but the major improvement came after 25 treatments and more significantly after 40. I continue the treatments on a limited basis now to maintain the return of my health. I am so grateful to have learned about Edna and her light chamber; it has brought me back to life to enjoy my retirement!"

Conclusion

Douglas, I know you don't remember much of your treatment journey because you were in so much pain and deep depression. But for me and you, Doug, those months were filled with the highest quality time we spent together through our entire relationship. I wrote this book to serve others out of serving you and what a blessing it has been. But I also wrote this book for you. I wanted you to hear your story and stand proud. Since you relied on me for all of your needs, you learned the importance of nutrition, hydration, detoxification and emotional health. You learned the value of natural remedies and now better understand my work with hyperbaric oxygen, light and vibration therapy. You now value my love for service to others who suffer and you share in my mission. Thank you for committing, showing up, diving into the light, eating right, detoxing, exercising and loving yourself unconditionally. That is a recipe for extraordinary healing and a beautiful life!

Resources

April Koch, "The Nature of Light: Origin, Spectrum & Color Frequency." study.com. Accessed June 24, 2017. http://study.com/academy/lesson/the-nature-of-light-origin-spectrum-color-frequency.html.

WebMD, "Causes of Stress." webmd.com. Accessed June 24, 2017. http://www.webmd.com/balance/guide/causes-of-stress.

Dr. Mercola, "Are Saunas Good for Your Brain?" mercola.com. Accessed June 24, 2017. http://articles.mercola.com/sites/articles/archive/2017/01/12/sauna-health-benefits.aspx.

Dr. Mercola, "Exercise is an Important Part of Cancer Prevention and Care." Mercola.com. Accessed June 24, 2017. http://

fitness.mercola.com/sites/fitness/archive/2017/03/24/exercise-benefits-for-cancer.aspx.

Addiction Blog, "The Efficiency of Hyperbaric Oxygen Therapy (HBOT) in Addiction Treatment." addictionblog. org. Accessed June 24, 2017. http://addictionblog.org/ treatment/the-efficacy-of-hyperbaric-oxygen-therapy-hbot-in-addiction-treatment/.

Burke, Ph. D. Dr. Tom. "Nitric Oxide Series, Part Nine: How Light (Photo Energy) May Increase Local NO and Vasodilation." Diabetes In Control. A free weekly diabetes newsletter for Medical Professionals. September 22, 2015. Accessed June 23, 2017. http://www.diabetesincontrol. com/nitric-oxide-series-part-nine-how-light-photo-energy-may-increase-local-no-and-vasodilation/.

Joseph Mercola, "How a High-Fat Diet Helps Starve Cancer" LewRockwell.com. Accessed June 23, 2017. https://www. lewrockwell.com/2016/05/joseph-mercola/cancer-cells-love-sugar/.

Mayo Clinic Staff, "Cancer survivors: Care for your body after treatment..."mayoclinic.org, Accessed June 24, 2017. http://www.mayoclinic.org/diseases-conditions/cancer/in-depth/cancer-survivor/ART-20044015

Dr. Nicholas Gonzales, "Dr. Gonzalez Dismantles the Ketogenic Diet for Cancer." chrisbeatcancer.com. Accessed June

23, 2017. http://www.chrisbeatcancer.com/dr-gonzalez-dismantles-ketogenic-diet-for-cancer/.

Edward Lucarini, "HBOT treatment for patients with Alcoholism, Drug Addiction, and Narcotic Addiction in Post-Intoxication & Abstinence Period." hbot.com. Accessed June 23, 2017. http://www.hbot.com/blog/edward-lucarini/hbot-treatment-patients-alcoholism-drug-addiction-and-narcotic-addiction-post-i.

"Hospital-Based Hyperbaric Facilities." hyperbariclink.com. Accessed June 23, 2017. https://www.hyperbariclink.com/hyperbaric-oxygen-therapy/hospital-hyperbaric-treatment-centers.aspx.

"Hyperbaric Oxygen Therapy." nwhospital.org,. Accessed June 23, 2017. http://nwhospital.org/medical-services/hyperbaric-oxygen-therapy/.

"Hyperbaric Oxygen Therapy." Naturopathic Doctor News and Review. Accessed June 23, 2017. http://ndnr.com/anti-aging/hyperbaric-oxygen-therapy/.

Lucas, Jim. "What Is Infrared?" livescience.com March 26, 2015. Accessed June 24, 2017. https://www.livescience.com/50260-infrared-radiation.html.

Selected Abstracts, Citations and Case Studies, "Mechanisms of Action for Infrared Light on Tissue Healing." alternativeworldwidehealth.com Accessed June 23,

2017. http://www.alternativeworldwidehealth.com/files/Articles%20for%20linking/Mechanisms_of_Action_for_Infrared_Light_on_Tissue_Healing.pdf

Dr. Sungkyoo Lim, PhD, "NASA Light Therapy NIR & LED." shinewithlight.com. Accessed June 23, 2017. http://shinewithlight.com/wp-content/uploads/2013/04/NASA-research-article.pdf

"Coping with Nerve Damage (Neuropathy)." cancercare.org. Accessed June 24, 2017. http://www.cancercare.org/publications/215-coping_with_nerve_damage_neuropathy.

"Peripheral Neuropathy - Topic Overview." webmd.com Accessed June 24, 2017. http://www.webmd.com/brain/tc/peripheral-neuropathy-topic-overview.

"Physical Activity and Cancer." cancer.gov. Accessed June 24, 2017. https://www.cancer.gov/about-cancer/causes-prevention/risk/obesity/physical-activity-fact-sheet.

Harvard Women's Health Watch, "Anxiety and physical illness." health.harvard.edu. Accessed June 24, 2017. http://www.health.harvard.edu/staying-healthy/anxiety_and_physical_illness.

"Scientific Basis of Coffee Enemas - Gerson Institute." Accessed June 24, 2017. https://gerson.org/pdfs/How_Coffee_Enemas_Work.pdf

Seyfried, Thomas N., and Laura M. Shelton. "Cancer as a metabolic disease." nutritionandmetabolism. biomedcentral.com. January 27, 2010. Accessed June 23, 2017. https://nutritionandmetabolism.biomedcentral.com/articles/10.1186/1743-7075-7-7.

Sukoff, M. H. "Effects of hyperbaric oxygenation." Journal of neurosurgery. September 2001. Accessed June 23, 2017. https://www.ncbi.nlm.nih.gov/pubmed/11565887/.

Dr. Joseph Mercola, "Dr. Joseph Mercola on an easy way to detox and heal your body"

lewrockwell.com. Accessed June 24, 2017. https://www.lewrockwell.com/2015/07/joseph-mercola/sweat-it-out-2/.

TV, Recharge. "E-Motion: The Movie." E-Motion. Accessed June 24, 2017. http://www.e-motionthemovie.com/.

"What are the benefits of alkaline foods for cancer patients?" reference.com. Accessed June 23, 2017. https://www.reference.com/health/benefits-alkaline-foods-cancer-patients-bec2c09f041015b9.

Acknowledgements

First and foremost I am so thankful to God for this wonderful gift. It was His vision, His plan and His execution. There is no one else who could have orchestrated such a beautiful outcome. Thank you dear Lord for your blessings.

Secondly, I want to thank my husband for choosing to live and for choosing to love more fully. Thank you Douglas for encouraging me to share our story even though you are a private man. My heart swells with love, pride and gratitude when I think of what you have been through and where you are now. Thank you for nurturing your compassionate side and opening your heart to helping others in need of healing. I love you with all my heart. These will be the best years of our lives together!

I thank my mother and father for giving me a servants' heart and for loving me unconditionally. I feel you smiling down on me with pride. Out of all five of your children you probably never imagined I would be an author. I love you and miss you both.

This book would not have been possible without the loving support of our family and friends. I thank you all for your encouragement, love, care and patience through this journey. I am especially grateful to Meeka, Kiira and Maree who put their lives on hold to be our daily support team. I am also extremely grateful to Caitlin for keeping our business open in my extended absence and to Jamie for stepping out of his comfort zone to keep the hyperbaric clients happy and cared for. Thank you for taking time out of your busy lives to help us during our darkest times. We love you all so much.

Doug and I found ourselves in a critical situation. Doug would not have lived and I would not have been able to write this book without the help of these extraordinary people, whom I especially want to thank:

Dr. A, for saving Doug's life. We were so blessed to have found you. The empathy you showed Doug on our first visit was such a gift, we knew he was in the hands of someone who truly cared and was willing to fight for him. Thank you for working overtime and for being so talented, meticulous, genuine and humble. We appreciate you and are forever grateful.

Angela; you are more than a nurse; you are an angel. You gave me strength when I needed it, you comforted me when I could not contain my tears and my fears and you empowered me with knowledge to be a better caregiver. From the very first day you treated Doug like he was your only patient and that his life mattered. Thank you for being our angel.

Dr. B for jumping through hoops with Dr. A to save Doug's life; for convincing the hospital to allow his chemotherapy to be administered as an inpatient at midnight. Thank you for being so gracious, calm and confident; that was what we needed in our time of crisis. We were so honored and blessed to have such a beautiful, intelligent and tender oncologist on Doug's team. Thank you from the bottom of our hearts.

Mark Matthias, Ali Novinger and the staff at Beaches restaurant for going above and beyond; from making Doug's special soup behind the scenes and to sending food our way no matter how far away we were. You guys are amazing!

Dr. Rose Paisley, ND, for your patience, guidance and knowledge. You have a special talent. You were truly a lifeline following treatment and so tender with my husband. Thank you for your persistence.

Connie Burgstahler, LMP, who kept urging me to write this book when I continued to have every excuse not to. I thank you for gently pushing me to share our story. More than anything, thank you for all the time you spent breaking down the scar tissue in Doug's neck while the radiation was still burning.

Dr. Heather Boyd-Roberts for all of the knowledge and kindness you bestowed upon me over the many years of working together. It was that knowledge that guided me through those dark days of caregiving and I credit much of his healing to the natural remedies I learned from you. I am forever grateful to you Heather.

Krista Ernsdorf, PT, for getting Doug moving when he didn't want to and for being tough and tender at the same time.

Anna Axland for kicking his butt Monday and Wednesday mornings for the last year and on-going to regain strength, mobility, flexibility and posture. You are a dream; we appreciate you so much.

Angela Lauria for your beautiful bold vision of using your message to make a difference and to serve others; for helping me know that it is not how well you write, it is having a servant's heart and getting the book done that matters. Thank you for being brutally honest with me and pushing me through to completion. You are one of a kind, consistent and brilliant! Thank you for showing up that way. I love you for being you!

To the Morgan James Publishing team: Special thanks to David Hancock, CEO & Founder for believing in me and my message. To my Author Relations Manager, Margo Toulouse, thanks for making the process seamless and easy. Many more thanks to everyone else, but especially Jim Howard, Bethany Marshall and Nickcole Watkins.

About the Author

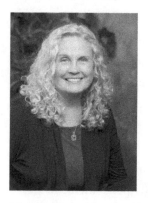

Edna has over a decade of experience as a Naturopathic Physician Assistant in addition to five years as a Therapeutic Esthetician. She is a graduate of the Euro Institute of Holistic Skin Care and is a certified technician for Nambudipad's Allergy Elimination Techniques (NAET) allergy treatments, LED and Infrared Light Therapy, Heart Rate Variability and other healing techniques. Edna also facilitated classes for the American Cancer Society at Adventist Hospital for six years.

She received her certification from the International Hyperbaric Association for the application of Mild Hyperbaric Oxygen Therapy (MHBOT). Her training, education and personal, professional and practical application of both light and MHBOT therapies provide unparalleled insight into the treatment of her clients for pain management and healing.

Her passion to help suffering clients achieve wellness is a product of her own personal journey through pain, injuries and disease, which has shaped her into a compassionate healer. This journey reached its pinnacle when she was called upon to nurse her husband through late stage, nearly terminal throat cancer. Her most recent passion was the result of the extraordinary healing he experienced after chemotherapy and radiation. She loves helping other cancer patients find hope in their journey to achieving a faster and more complete healing and a higher quality of life.

Edna is a native of Colorado and moved to Vancouver, Washington nearly 20 years ago. She and her husband Doug have three sons and four daughters (triplets included), five grandchildren and three aquatic turtles. She is truly blessed.

Blessings to You

Thank you for taking the time to read this book. It is my wish that the information will assist you in your healing journey.

The quality of your life moving forward is up to you. Opening your mind to natural remedies and alternative treatments is just the beginning. Taking action will make the difference you desire and give you a higher quality of life.

If you feel the need for guidance, I invite you to schedule a free consultation with me. We can discuss your unique situation, I will share the "10 Most Important Tips for Healing" and as a special gift to lift you up I will send you my favorite inspirational cards of HOPE!

Are you ready to heal? I would love to help you. Please contact me by filling out the form at:ChemoAndRadiationRecovery.com.

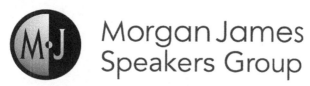

Morgan James
Speakers Group

We connect Morgan James published
authors with live and online events
and audiences who will benefit
from their expertise.

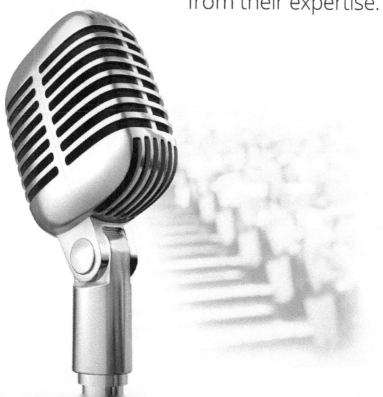

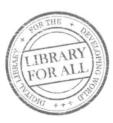

Morgan James makes all of our titles available
through the Library for All Charity Organization.

www.LibraryForAll.org

Printed in the USA
CPSIA information can be obtained
at www.ICGtesting.com
JSHW082357140824
68134JS00020B/2120

9 781683 508212